Professional Communication in Speech-Language Pathology

How to Write, Talk, and Act Like a Clinician

Second Edition

Professional Communication in Speech-Language Pathology

How to Write, Talk, and Act Like a Clinician

Second Edition

A. Embry Burrus
Laura B. Willis

PLURAL
PUBLISHING
INC.
SAN DIEGO
OXFORD
MELBOURNE

5521 Ruffin Road
San Diego, CA 92123

e-mail: info@pluralpublishing.com
Web site: http://www.pluralpublishing.com

ISBN-13: 978-1-59756-505-9
ISBN-10: 1-59756-505-9
Library of Congress Control Number: 2012952517

Contents

Preface

Let us tell you about Liz, a composite of hundreds of undergraduate students who have passed through our training program. Liz was a sophomore who sat in the front row of the language acquisition class. She sported a pair of denim jeans with large holes in the knees and ragged edges around the ankles, a T-shirt that advertised an oyster bar in Pensacola, Florida, dark purple lipstick, and a diamond-studded nose ring. Her hair was jet black with a highlighted strand of hot pink framing her face. She was a warm and friendly student who wanted, more than anything else, to help children with autism. What was evident at the time, however, was the vast distance she needed to travel to make her dreams a reality. How could this Liz, who had no clue about the nature of professional service delivery, become "professional" Liz the speech-language pathologist who works in a community clinic, school system, or medical facility? If Liz did not get some instruction in professional appearance, professional demeanor, and professional communication before practicum started, her initial clinical experience would be like diving into a very cold pool of water. It is for this reason that most universities have a course with a title such as "Introduction to Clinical Practicum" that spells out in painful detail the rules, regulations, and behaviors associated with being a professional clinician. Make no mistake, the metamorphosis from student to professional clinician was not easy for Liz, and she hit a few rough patches along the way. Fortunately, however, the end of Liz's story is a happy one. Through 3 years of practicum experience in later undergraduate and graduate studies, she gradually learned to project herself as a professional and now is working as a certified speech-language pathologist in a large children's hospital. This book is designed to make the journey from student to clinician more predictable and a bit less onerous for students like Liz.

Preparing a student for the clinical practicum experience has always been a challenge. The students come to us eager about embarking on a new and exciting profession. They have studied some of the disorders of communication in classes and seen videotapes of treatment sessions performed either by master clinicians in the field or more advanced graduate students. When the time for clinical practicum arrives, they are enthusiastic and worried about their first foray into a clinical relationship. Unfortunately, clinical work is one of those enterprises that almost all students enter with no practical experience. By our calculations, people in the speech-language pathology major have about 3 years to complete the transition from carefree undergraduate student to concerned clinical professional with a master's degree.

We asked ourselves many questions in planning this text: *Wouldn't it be nice if we could forewarn students about common pitfalls in the clinical practicum process, so these could be avoided? Would the student operate more efficiently in off-campus placements if we spent a little time introducing the nature of those settings before the student leaves the university environment? Would clinical reports be of higher quality if we gave examples and provided suggestions for writing and a list of common errors? Would the students be less anxious if we prepared them ahead of time with examples of the clinical documentation used in medical and school settings? Would the student be better able to verbally interact with clients, families, other professionals, and supervisors if we provided suggestions regarding professional verbal communication?* Clearly, we felt that the answers to our questions would no doubt be in the affirmative.

This textbook was designed to help beginning speech-language pathology students as they approach the clinical practicum experience. There are several major themes that weave their way through the text. First, we wanted to provide the student with a sense of professional demeanor common to speech-language pathologists. It is our view that such professionalism is largely communicated through our interactions. For instance, a person's behavior, written communications, and verbal communications are perceived by others as significant indices of professionalism. Actions can include such varied components as appearance, ethical behavior, decision-making, planning clinical work, and nonverbal communication skills. Actions, as they say, often speak louder than words. Written communications range from various clinical reports to progress notes and professional correspondence. We project our professionalism every time we write any type of clinical documentation. Verbal communication with clients, families, other professionals, and supervisors is the means by which we provide information, obtain information, counsel, and solve problems related to clinical activity. Because the features of professional behavior, professional writing, and professional speaking are so important to defining a professional, we elected to name this book *Professional Communication in Speech-Language Pathology: How to Write, Talk, and Act Like a Clinician*. In this second edition of the text, we have revised, updated, and expanded upon the original text to include up to date research and current trends in clinical practicum.

A second theme of this book involves practicum settings. Since clinical practicum is different from any other experience these students have encountered, it is important to provide a road map of where they are headed in the process of learning to be a competent clinician. For this reason, we have chosen to discuss three practicum settings in almost every chapter: (a) university clinics, (b) medical settings, and (c) public school settings. The chapters provide examples of professional written communication that are unique to each type of workplace. Clinical documentation is similar yet different across these work settings and students should be aware of those similarities and differences before they experience an off-campus placement. But the information in this text goes beyond paperwork. For example, we discuss professional verbal communication in dealing with clients, families, other professionals, and supervisors across work settings as well.

A third component in almost every chapter is our delineation of proactive suggestions that are helpful to the student in navigating the various settings of clinical practicum. In this way, the book serves as a kind of survival guide to clinical practicum because we discuss common pitfalls across settings and ways to avoid them. If we expect students to perform well across different practicum experiences, then we should tell them how their behavior and documentation should change in these settings as compared to the university clinic. In many cases, it is as simple as just listing things to do and not do. Ironically, many of the pitfalls in practicum settings are caused by poor communication. Fortunately, it is also professional communication that plays a major role in solving practicum difficulties.

The final characteristic of this book is that we attempted to write it in a student-friendly style with copious examples and vignettes to help the student understand the material not only intellectually, but on an emotional level as well. Many books on clinical practicum are compilations of rules, references, regulations, and writing exercises that, while certainly important, are often difficult to digest. This book generally discusses most of these issues, but also illustrates them in a practical and interesting way. We hope the text can be useful as part of a course that introduces students to the exciting arena of clinical practicum.

SECTION I

Introduction to Professional Communication, Clinical Practicum Sites, and Ethics

1 The Nature of Professionalism and Professional Communication

INTRODUCTION

The field of speech-language pathology is one of the most respected of the helping professions. Speech-language pathologists (SLPs) work in a variety of settings with a cross-section of the population and a diverse group of related professionals. When we think of the word *professional*, what does this really mean? Webster's Dictionary defines *professional* as "[p]ertaining to a profession or to a calling; as professional studies, pursuits, duties, engagements; professional character or skill." The definition implies that there are certain characteristics of a professional that not only include duties (e.g., assessment and treatment in the case of the SLP), but also interactions (engagements) and personal attributes (character or skill.) Typically, a person knows if the treatment being received is professional and can easily distinguish unprofessional behavior on the part of a service provider. Yet explaining what it means to act as a professional may be as elusive as capturing lightning in a bottle. It is not difficult to recognize unprofessional demeanor, as illustrated by this account by Joseph Snyder, a businessman who is suffering from depression:

> Dr. Murphy's address on Mimosa Street turned out to be an old hotel populated by unsavory looking characters who sat on the rickety front porch. I found Dr. Murphy in the telephone book under "professional counseling services," which I was seeking for my depression. I had to wake the desk clerk who directed me to room 112 and I knocked on the door. A loud voice from inside the room yelled, "COME IN." I opened the door to reveal a middle-aged man sitting in a dilapidated recliner wearing an old Oriental bathrobe and sipping on an umbrella drink.

> Surrounding the chair were old newspapers and fast food containers that had been there for weeks. Upon seeing me he said, "What's up?" It was clear to me immediately that professionalism is not conferred on a person by a simple listing in the telephone book.

The extreme example above illustrates lack of professionalism on many levels. The next day, Joe Snyder tells us of his second attempt at finding help:

> The entrance to Dr. Estrada's office was a stained glass doorway between two large potted palm trees. The waiting room was lit by bright sunlight, furnished with striped wing chairs and had mahogany tables containing carefully arranged magazines. Behind a counter sat a receptionist who wore a blue silk dress and a smile. I approached the receptionist and told her that I had a nine o'clock appointment with Dr. Estrada. She said, "Please have a seat in the waiting room. Dr. Estrada will be right with you." In about five minutes, Dr. Estrada appeared, shook my hand and said, "I'm Dr. James Estrada and it's nice to meet you, Mr. Snyder." Then I was invited into Dr. Estrada's private office. It was a large, wood-paneled room that included a library of books and journals, several framed diplomas and licenses on the wall, and a number of decorative plants. After we were seated, Dr. Estrada said, "Let's get started by having you tell me what brings you in to see me today." As I began to tell my story, I could not help but think that this was the way it was supposed to be.

The overall difference between these two vignettes could be described in terms of physical appearances of the offices, demeanor of the office staff, and the language used by the psychologists. However, an overall discriminating variable between the two scenarios is the construct of professionalism. In one situation, professional behavior was lacking and in the other it was not. Again, we know professionalism when we see it, but it is difficult to exactly quantify. That is probably because being professional involves many variables that all interact in complex ways.

According to Brehm et al. (2006), the notion of professionalism is not monolithic and is in fact composed of multiple components. One component of professionalism includes professional parameters such as ethical and legal issues that guide many aspects of clinical practice. A second component of professionalism is professional behavior, which includes "discipline-related knowledge and skills, appropriate relationships with clients and colleagues, and acceptable appearance and attitudes" (p. 1). The final ingredient in professionalism is "responsibility to the profession and to oneself, clients, employers, and community" (p. 1). Thus, the combination of professional parameters, professional behavior, and professional responsibility form the core of professionalism in any field.

Although the scenarios at the beginning of this chapter came from the field of psychology, the various aspects of professionalism could have been illustrated using many different fields. The literature from many health-related disciplines is concerned with professionalism both at the level of training programs and in the clinical practice after graduation. For example, fields such as medicine (American Academy of Pediatrics, 2007), occupational therapy (Randolph, 2003), pharmacy (Hammer, Berger, & Beardsley, 2003), and nursing (Clooman, Davis, & Burnett, 1999) all view professionalism as a critical variable in clinical practice and in training programs. But it is not only in so-called "white collar" positions that professionalism is important. Even in jobs that are technically not "professional" we have certain standards of demeanor that are expected. For example, when you take your car in for repair you expect a certain degree of professionalism from the employees. We expect restaurant employees to behave professionally when serving customers. Professional behavior is an important part of every job from plumbing and carpentry to lawn maintenance and selling of automobiles. In all of these fields we expect the practitioners to have certain knowledge and skills that allow them to competently perform the job and we expect to be treated with respect. If these expectations are not met, people tend to not return for additional services.

It should be no surprise to students that professionalism is an important and critical component in the practice of speech-language pathology. When clients and other professionals deal with the SLP, there are certain expectations for professionalism. The general public expects an SLP to work in a physical setting that instills confidence in clients and represents the professional as someone to be respected as a clinician. The language we use with clients and people from other disciplines should be professional in tone and content. The reports we generate in the course of assessment and treatment of patients should reflect the professionalism of our field. Professionalism is not just about how clients and other disciplines perceive us; it is also about how it makes others feel about themselves. If you treat a client with professionalism, empathy, and respect, it will create an environment that is conducive to positive clinical change. Hegde and Davis (2010) discuss how professionalism manifests itself in SLP for practicum students:

[G]eneral rules of professional behavior include punctuality in meeting clinical appointments and clinic deadlines; working cooperatively with office staff, supervisors, and other student clinicians; assuming responsibility for clinic equipment and clinic facilities; being well-prepared for each clinical session; and maintaining appropriate dress and demeanor. Professional demeanor is one of the initial factors on which a student clinician is evaluated. Professional demeanor is a vague term, but refers to such behaviors as appearing confident in your abilities, communicating clearly and appropriately with the client and supervisor, presenting yourself as a mature adult, following prescribed rules and effectively utilizing clinical time. (p. 68)

You can see that professionalism is not only expected of seasoned clinicians but of clinicians in training as well. One objective of this book is to help students realize the importance of professionalism in becoming an SLP and how one's behavior, language, and writing are important factors in becoming a professional.

One common thread running through the concept of professionalism is the idea that it is demonstrated largely through various forms of communication. The physical properties of a clinical environment communicate important information about professionalism as illustrated in the psychology examples on the previous page. Nonverbal communication can indicate confidence and expertise as well as empathy for the client. Verbal communication with clients and other professionals can be a clear indication of a clinician's knowledge about the field, empathy, and ability to perform assessment and treatment activities. Finally, written communication (e.g., letters, reports, treatment plans, progress notes) represents the clinician to others when face-to-face interactions are not possible. The notion of communication is inseparable from the construct of professionalism. It is how professionalism manifests itself to clients and other professionals. Thus, it is not simply a coincidence that we have used the term *professional communication* in the title of this textbook. The term is very broad and includes both written as well as verbal interactions. Figure 1–1 shows examples of professional communication that represent the written and verbal modalities. Although we will be spending more time on the written forms of professional communication, it is important to touch on verbal communication as well. Let us spend a little time discussing the types of professional communication illustrated in Figure 1–1. In subsequent chapters of the present text we cover each of these areas in more detail.

PROFESSIONAL WRITTEN COMMUNICATION

Both students and professionals are required to generate professional documents related to evaluations, treatment planning, and treatment reporting. Figure 1–1 shows several important areas of professional written communication:

1. **Diagnostic reports:** These are clinical reports that summarize the results of an evaluation including standardized and nonstandardized testing of a client who has received a formal assessment of his communication abilities. The diagnostic report becomes part of a patient's clinical record and is often transmitted, with client permission, to other professionals. Our reports represent not only the student who wrote them, but the student's clinical supervisor and the facility (university, hospital, school system) that performed the assessment.

2. **Daily treatment plans:** Students in training are often required to develop written goals and procedures in the form of a treatment plan that is submitted to the clinical supervisor for review and approval. The treatment plan outlines the plan for the therapy session with regard to goals and procedures. Students may also be asked to include rationales from theory or research for goal selection and the use of particular procedures in the treatment plan. The treatment plan should represent the result of considerable thought by the student after reviewing the case information, appropriate textbooks, and class notes on the appropriate disorder, and discussions with the clinical supervisor.

3. **Treatment reports:** These reports are designed to summarize the progress of a client in a treatment program and address changes in client behavior on goals and objectives of therapy over a period of time. These reports become part of a client's file and serve to communicate the treatment approach and progress to other professionals or future students who will work with the case in subsequent semesters. For example, a client being seen in the university clinic may also be seen in the public schools and treatment reports are routinely sent to the SLP in the school system to make him or her aware of the client's progress at the university.

4. **Progress notes:** Progress notes are short synopses written on a daily or weekly basis and kept in a client's working file or hospital chart to summarize the client's performance and progress toward short-term goals and objectives. These notes may be read by other professionals in school or medical settings as a way of communicating client progress in many areas.

5. **Professional correspondence:** These are letters written to referral sources, parents, family members, or other professionals discussing general

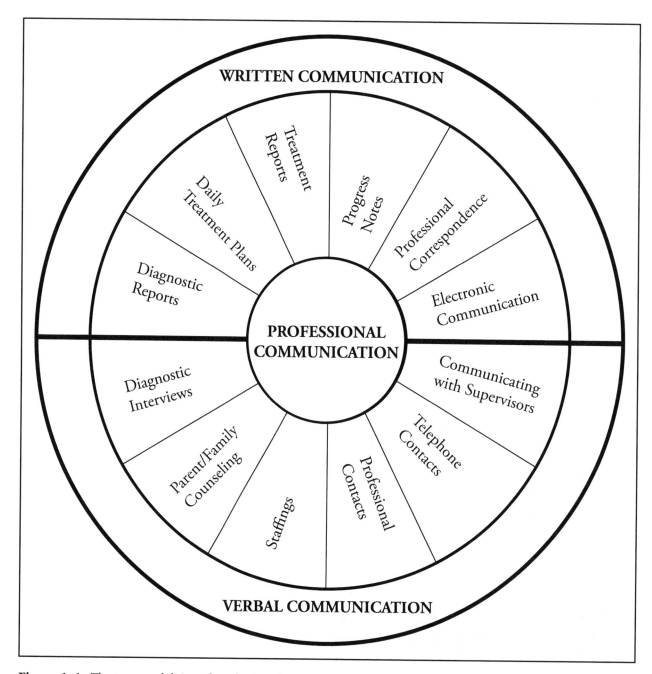

Figure 1–1. The two modalities of professional communication.

clinical matters or clinical issues related to a particular patient. Sometimes this correspondence is as simple as expressing appreciation for a referral from another professional. For instance, a physician may refer a patient with vocal nodules for voice therapy to the university clinic. It is always important to thank other professionals for referrals so that a good working relationship is maintained. You might also write a letter to a physician to whom you are referring a patient from the university clinic. There are many different types of clinical correspondence and it is important that each be handled in a professional manner.

6. **Electronic communication:** The use of electronic mail or facsimile machines is sometimes used to relate clinical information to other professionals. Although we do not typically send reports via e-mail, it is important that any correspondence with other professionals or clients be done in as professional a manner as possible. It is not unusual for reports to be faxed between clinical settings, but as in any electronic communication, the importance of maintaining confidentiality of client information is paramount. For example, sending a report via fax relinquishes control over who receives it. There are some reports that temporary office workers should not have access to.

In all six areas mentioned above, the SLP is expected to adhere to specific professional guidelines regarding types of language used, protection of confidential information, and format requirements. The guidelines are similar across the six forms of professional written communication, but there are also subtle differences. These guidelines are discussed in more detail in later chapters of this text.

In all settings, you should acknowledge that the clinical record is a communication tool that is shared among a group of professionals, all of whom serve the client. This team may include teachers, therapists, physicians, psychologists, and other medical professionals. It always includes the patient and their family or caregivers. The record, which includes your reports, is a representation of the quality of service you provide and is vital for others to reference when determining what is best for the client. Paul (1994) cites the following as purposes of documentation:

- Justification of treatment
- Support diagnosis and treatment (including medical necessity and need for skilled services)
- Describe client progress
- Describe client response to interventions
- Justify discharge from treatment
- Support reimbursement
- Communicate with other professionals
- Justify clinical decisions

- Document communication among involved parties (practitioners, client, caregivers, or legally responsible parties)
- Protect legal interests of client, service provider, and facility
- Serve as evidence in a court of law
- Provide data for research (i.e., efficacy)

You might be asking yourself, "How difficult can it be to learn how to write all these different kinds of documents?" You may have been an excellent student in English composition, but unfortunately, clinical writing is quite different from generating a term paper or short story. In professional writing you will be expected to use professional terminology, write the document in the appropriate format, and employ very specific descriptions of a client's performance in reporting assessment or treatment results. You might be saying, "Why can't I just write it my way instead of using all these technical terms and strange formats?" Failure to understand the importance of clinical writing as a unique genre has led, on more than one occasion, to poor grades in clinical practicum. It is important for you to realize early on that clinical supervisors take professional written communication *very* seriously. Professional writing or reporting is *always* included on clinical practicum grading forms and students are evaluated on the punctuality of submitting paperwork, the quality of their professional writing, the completeness of the reports, and the appropriateness of the paperwork for the work setting. Ironically, although students are certain to be evaluated on these important facets of clinical ability, there is often little direct classroom teaching that focuses on professional writing. Textbooks most often devote a single chapter or part of a chapter to professional writing, and this is typically not enough exposure to prepare students for different types of reports (e.g., evaluation, treatment) or paperwork peculiar to a specific work setting (e.g., IEP/IFSP in schools, progress notes in medical settings, etc.).

How, then, do students learn professional writing skills if not in classes or textbook chapters? The reality is that students generally learn professional writing through the grim experience of generating a report for a clinical supervisor and then bearing witness to the supervisor figuratively "shredding" their work by slashing through the paragraphs with a red felt-tipped marker. In addition to the deleted utterances, the supervisor typically adds words and sometimes entire paragraphs with circles and arrows directing the student's attention even to the back of the page. Other supervisors merely make cryptic ciphers indicating that the student should "add more information," though not indicating how this should be done. This will lead to a second session of multicolored criticisms if the student cannot divine the intent of the supervisor. Students have also said that report writing style varies considerably by supervisor, and that what might be perfectly acceptable for one person may not be acceptable for another. An additional difficulty occurs when the student leaves the insulated setting of the university clinic for off-campus practicum. The student will soon learn that in the "real world," evaluation, treatment, and report writing are quite different from what goes on at the university. As such, students are buffeted about from one supervisor to another and one setting to another, and finally they "learn" professional writing through a process that involves much trial and error and some bruising of their egos. The present authors feel that professional writing is somewhat of a mystery to beginning students. We find it paradoxical that students are expected to learn professional writing largely through trial and error and with precious few resources that adequately address professional writing issues. This is precisely why we feel that a more proactive approach needs to be taken to professional writing in the form of a guidebook that is specifically directed to students in training. It is our hope that such a resource will demystify professional writing, illustrate appropriate formats used across work settings, discuss common errors that students tend to make, and show students examples of all the types of paperwork they will encounter at the upper undergraduate and graduate levels of their training. It is not possible to totally eliminate the frustrations associated with report writing for both students and supervisors because there is a certain amount of trial and error that *must* be experienced to learn this elusive craft. It is not necessary, however, to leave the entire process to chance. If we can provide explicit information in terms of report formats, typical writing errors, and professional language, the student can be more proactive and produce an initial effort that is closer to the desired target.

PROFESSIONAL VERBAL COMMUNICATION

The bottom portion of Figure 1–1 illustrates that professional communication is not confined to the written modality. There are many occasions on which students are expected to communicate verbally with parents, family members, or other professionals both in person and over the telephone. You might be thinking, "I already know how to talk to people. What is different about talking to people in a clinical setting?" Again, there is a certain professional demeanor and use of language that is expected in a clinical setting. There are certain terms to use, just as in clinical reports. There is even a "format" for what to talk about in certain situations. We briefly mention the areas of verbal professional communication below:

1. **Diagnostic interviews:** No matter what type of client you see in a diagnostic evaluation, the interaction always begins with an interview. In the context of the diagnostic interview you will be interested in controlling the conversation so that you can obtain information, give information, and explain the assessment results to the client/family (Haynes & Pindzola, 2012). These interviews require organization, planning, and skill that few people innately possess, and prowess comes with practice. Later in the text we talk more about professional communication in diagnostic interviews. For now, however, it is enough to realize that professional communication involves talking as well as writing.

2. **Parent/family counseling:** There are many occasions when we talk to parents and family members about diagnoses, treatment progress, referrals, or enlisting their help with the therapy program. Again, there are specific ways to communicate about such issues.

3. **Staffings:** In many work settings, a variety of professionals from different disciplines gather around a table together to discuss a particular client. For example, it would not be unusual to see a staffing that included an SLP, psychologist, classroom teacher, parent, and occupational therapist. Each professional contributes unique information to the staffing and is expected to

communicate professionally. There are guidelines for professional communication in such settings and we discuss these in later sections.

4. **Professional contacts:** In some cases the SLP will be asked to talk with physicians, physical therapists, radiologists, psychologists, teachers, special educators, and other professionals about a case. Although these are informal contacts, they still have the aura of professional communication.

5. **Telephone contacts:** Everything from scheduling cases for assessment and treatment to making referrals of a client to another professional often requires talking on the telephone. Again, professional verbal communication is critical.

6. **Communicating with supervisors:** As a student, you will have many opportunities to communicate with clinical supervisors, special education coordinators, directors of SLP in medical settings, principals of schools, and other

people to whom you have to answer for your activities. Professional verbal communication is important in all of these situations. You may be explaining the progress of a particular case or lobbying for monetary support to purchase tests and materials. Professional verbal communication is a key ingredient.

SHARED COMPONENTS OF PROFESSIONAL WRITTEN AND VERBAL COMMUNICATION

Figure 1–2 shows some shared components of professional written and verbal communication. By shared components, we mean that certain commonalities exist between the written and verbal expressions of professional communication. In many ways these components help to differentiate professional

Figure 1–2. Shared components of profession written and verbal communication.

communication from a typical conversational chat. We briefly discuss each below:

1. **Professional terminology:** In both verbal and written professional communication it is expected that appropriate terminology will be used by the SLP. We use terms such as *oral cavity* instead of *mouth* or *phonemes* instead of *sounds*. The SLP will discuss syntax, semantics, pragmatics, and morphology when talking about language. In both verbal and written interactions professional terms are appropriate to use, depending on the audience. As we discuss later, the context of communication in terms of where you are talking and to whom you are talking is important to consider when using discipline-specific terminology.

2. **Accuracy of information:** It is assumed that any professional communication will contain accurate information, whether it is a verbal interaction or a clinical report. If a professional is asked how a child scored on a test, it would not be appropriate to say, "I think he scored in the 5th percentile, or maybe the 40th." If you can't remember the score, do not speculate. In a written report, we describe assessment and treatment information accurately using test scores and descriptions of behavior because we do not want to say something without reliable evidence. Professionals always double-check the scoring and reporting of test data to ensure that it is accurate. There is typically a portion of a clinical report that allows a practitioner an opportunity to discuss "clinical impressions." This section of a report, however, is clearly demarcated from the parts of the writing that describe test scores and more objective information. Professional communication is highly concerned with accuracy.

3. **Organization:** Professional communication is usually orderly both in the written and verbal modalities. If you are part of a multidisciplinary staffing and are asked to talk about a child's language disorder and progress in treatment, the other professionals present do not expect you to embark on an unorganized stream of consciousness rant about the client. They expect you to provide some background information, talk a bit about assessment, outline the treatment goals, and discuss progress in therapy. Even though you are talking, there is a basic organization that is expected from a professional. Obviously, in clinical reports, there is a format that is unique to the work setting that guides your writing. Again, it is not like writing a letter home to your family, but a highly organized summary of very specific information written in professional language. Thus, organization is part of both written and verbal professional communication.

4. **Respect:** One of the hallmarks of professional communication involves showing respect for the client, family, or other professional. This is not merely a courtesy, but is demanded by the codes of ethics of virtually every professional organization. We must treat clients, families, and other professionals with respect as an ethical proscription. This is why we usually refer to adult clients as "Mr. Smith" or "Mrs. Jones" rather than "Charlie" or "Edith." Certainly, as a clinical relationship develops we may refer to clients by their first names, but only when it is mutually agreeable and appropriate. Respect is also shown when we take into account the feelings and attitudes of others in the course of our interactions. We do not want to offend clients or other professionals with either our reports or verbal interactions. We show respect when we listen to the opinions of other professionals about our clients and when we listen to our patients as they tell us about their struggles. In Chapter 11, we address interaction styles as they relate to patients of diverse cultural backgrounds. Respect is shown in the quality of our physical facilities, the comfort of the chairs, and the reading material provided in our waiting rooms. After all, making patients wait in the squalor of a filthy, disorganized waiting room is a sign of disrespect to our clients. If we show up at the clinic in a T-shirt and jeans, we are saying to our clients that we do not think enough of them to present a professional appearance.

5. **Objectivity:** Part of professional communication, whether verbal or in writing, is that it is unbiased and reflects objective reality as much as possible. We assume that the professional SLP will gather appropriate information in an assess-

ment and objectively interpret the data. Professional communication is not as much about a clinician's opinion as it is about evidence that can be documented. Professionals should never say something for which there is not adequate evidence or misrepresent the information that they are communicating. For instance, a clinician should not indicate that a child has cognitive limitations without the appropriate diagnosis. We would not want to indicate that a person has word retrieval difficulties without documenting this through assessment. For instance, if we said, "This child has behavior problems," it could be construed by the reader that he had actually been diagnosed with behavior disorder. It is much better to describe any behaviors that are of concern rather than provide inaccurate information.

6. **Sensitivity to context:** Contextual sensitivity affects professional communication in several ways. First, it is important to communicate in an appropriate way based on the setting in which the communication takes place. For example, in verbal communication in a hospital setting, certain words are used that are unique to that environment. One can use abbreviations such as *NICU, FIM scores, ADL, p.r.n.,* and *ROM*, and people in the medical setting will know what you are talking about. However, if you use these terms in the public school setting, teachers might not know what you mean. Conversely, in the school system you might use terms such as *Title I, Bloom's taxonomy, ESL, portfolio assessment,* and *IDEA*, which would be less understood in medical settings. At any rate, sensitivity to the context is an important influence on professional verbal communication. Context also has a large effect on professional written communication. For instance, the format for written reports and progress notes differs dramatically among university clinics, medical settings, and school environments. Your written communication must change depending on the context of the work setting. A second implication of sensitivity to context in professional communication concerns the person to whom you are talking or writing. For example, parents and caregivers are a very diverse group in terms of social status

and educational level. You cannot explain the results of an evaluation the same way to a person with a graduate degree and another person with an eighth grade education, yet you have to do it professionally in both cases. In written communication, reports tend to be written in professional language and would not be understandable by some parents. In these cases we send a "parent-friendly" summary letter that tells them the critical information in the report. When talking to other professionals, we must discriminate which terminology people from other disciplines may and may not understand and adjust our conversation appropriately. Similarly, if we are sending a report, incorporating terms specific to our discipline might make our report less understandable to someone from occupational therapy. Thus, professional verbal and written communication must change with the context in which we are communicating, both in terms of the setting and the person to whom we are talking.

How do students learn about professional verbal communication? This is an interesting question because there are typically no specific courses that deal with the issue. Most students learn how to communicate professionally by modeling clinical supervisors and watching students who are further along in their training. Watching the behavior of an experienced clinician who is communicating professionally goes a long way toward teaching less experienced students how to act in a clinical role. In most cases, beginning students are not given the responsibility to independently interview clients, meet with other professionals, or counsel families. Students usually start by observing such activities during their required hours of observation. When students receive their first clinical assignments, they typically are asked to conduct certain parts of interviews, staffing presentations, or counseling efforts, but do not have independent responsibility. A student progressing through the training program is given a greater role in professional verbal communication and any missteps are pointed out after the interaction by the clinical supervisor. A good strategy for any student in training is to take advantage of every opportunity to observe your clinical faculty engaged in professional communication with clients, families, or representatives of other disciplines.

In the upcoming chapters we discuss both written and verbal communication in more detail to provide students with some general guidelines that will help you navigate your training program. As you will see in the next chapter, there is no one way to write reports, nor is there just one format for verbal interaction.

2 Learning as They Change the Rules: The Many Faces of Clinical Practicum

University Supervisor: "Always dress up when you are working with clients."

Hospital Supervisor: "You can wear scrubs to work."

University Supervisor: "Your report was not long enough and did not have sufficient detail."

Hospital Supervisor: "Your report was far too long."

University Practicum Student: "My client has been coming to the clinic for five years . . . we call him a 'lifer'."

Hospital Practicum Student: "We see our patients in acute care for only a few days."

University Supervisor: "Always take a detailed case history and put it in your report."

Hospital Supervisor: "Our patients usually can't give a reliable case history. All we have is a couple of lines in the chart written by the case worker."

University Supervisor: "Administer standardized tests in their entirety according to the instruction manual so you can compare the scores to norms."

Hospital Supervisor: "We rarely give a complete standardized test. We have taken tasks from many tests and made up our own assessment protocol."

University Practicum Student: "We always have to remember to shred copies of our reports for confidentiality reasons."

Hospital Practicum Student: "We have gone paperless at the hospital and I use a computer to enter patient data."

University Practicum Student: "I got graded down because I didn't develop a home program for my client."

Skilled Nursing Practicum Student: "My patients will never go home, and no one comes to visit them."

University Practicum Student: "My client's spouse wants to talk after each session to learn how she can better help him find his words and improve his speech."

School Practicum Student: "We rarely see parents, except at IEP meetings once a year."

University Practicum Student: "My last report was five pages long."

School Practicum Student: "Our school has a software program to generate IEPs."

University Practicum Student: "I see this little boy individually and it's hard to develop enough activities for an hour session to keep him busy."

School Practicum Student: "I work mostly with kids in groups for less than half an hour."

University Practicum Student: "I have five goals I'm working on with my client; one is eye contact."

Hospital Practicum Student: "I have to be very careful how I write goals so we can bill for services."

University Practicum Student: "I'm working with a kid who substitutes w/r."

School Practicum Student: "In my school, kids with /r/ problems don't qualify for services."

University Practicum Student: "The client I work with brought me the sweetest thank-you note and my favorite cookies for working with him this semester."

Skilled Nursing Practicum Student: "Most of my patients have cognitive disorders and don't remember my name."

INTRODUCTION

The title of this chapter suggests that students in communication sciences and disorders will be confronted with many changes. On the surface, the statements from students and supervisors in the above box might seem in diametrical opposition. How can a clinical practice be acceptable to one student or supervisor on one occasion and unacceptable on another? Why is there such diversity in everything including clients, administrative procedures, opinions of supervisors, paperwork requirements, and types of therapy? The different perspectives illustrated above would seem to be a recipe for cognitive dissonance in our practicum students. Is it all part of an insidious plot to drive you completely insane? How can you be successful if the rules keep changing? Do not despair. We are here to help you.

If you are reading this book as part of your curriculum in communication sciences and disorders, we would like to welcome you to an exciting, diverse, and challenging profession. Over many years of teaching in a university training program, we have seen scores of students who decided to major in speech-language pathology. We have watched with great interest as they passed through the various phases of the curriculum and emerged on the other end as competent professionals. Through their training we saw the wonder on their faces as they began to understand the marvelous process of communication and all of the disorders that can rob a person of these critical abilities. We watched their first tentative therapy sessions and then saw them come strutting back from their internship showing all the confidence of a seasoned veteran. Over the course of training, however, we also were witness to many looks of consternation, confusion, and frustration as these students approached specific transition points in their programs. Much of their disquiet revolved more around the practicum experience than the coursework. Classes, after so long, become easy to deal with and students accepted into graduate programs usually have well-developed strategies for classroom success. Clinical practice, however, is a different matter. Here you are, after all those courses, actually working with someone for the first time. Let us assure you that everyone in this situation is uncertain, apprehensive, excited, and clueless. One of the things that make practicum so uncertain is that there is no one way to do it. If there were a magic formula for planning, executing, and reporting every disorder the same way, it would certainly be easier. But there are different types of clients, multiple disorders, varied supervisors, and diverse practicum settings, all of which make clinical work confusing to the novice therapist. Students have reported several specific sources of frustration with their practicum experiences over the years. First, they do not seem to understand how the university training program interfaces with other settings to form the overall practicum experience. Students do not seem to appreciate the "big picture" of why the university training program teaches certain things and why other settings may conduct business quite differently.

A second problem for students is making the adjustment between practicum settings as they go through clinical training. Each setting has a different type of caseload, physical characteristics, profes-

sionals, and requirements for clinical reporting. The student is buffeted between long narrative reports in the university clinic, chart notes in medical settings, and IEPs in school systems. Just when you reach a certain degree of comfort in one format, you are asked to perform therapy and clinical reporting in a completely different way. It is not that we are trying to drive you completely mad; there are logical reasons for these inconsistencies. Any accredited program in communication disorders must ensure that you obtain practicum experiences across different types of clinical environments. Thus, it should not be a surprise that you will be plucked from the comfortable venue of the university speech and hearing clinic and transplanted into a rehabilitation hospital in the space of just a semester. Your first reaction will no doubt be shock. Virtually everything is different, and even though you knew on some level that practicum sites would differ, you had no way to prepare yourself for such an abrupt transition. Our motivation behind writing this book was to help ease some of the transitions for students who are moved abruptly across different practicum settings. One of the most frustrating aspects of the changing terrain is the different paperwork requirements and professional behaviors that are required. We thought that if students could get a preview of the requirements across sites, the transitions would be a bit easier. That is why we have organized this book to some degree by work setting. So, if you are headed to a hospital next semester, check out the parts of the book that deal with reporting and behavior in medical settings. If you are assigned to a local elementary school, look at the sections devoted to educational settings. One thing is certain: each setting has its own unique culture and set of requirements for behavior and paperwork. Granted, you will not fully understand the nature of these things until you have spent a couple of weeks in a new practicum setting, but knowing a bit about what to expect will lessen your frustration and apprehension. The bulk of this book is concerned with professional communication across work settings, but we also provide some suggestions on how to survive as a practicum student in each workplace.

In the United States, there are approximately 250 training programs in SLP that are accredited by the American Speech-Language-Hearing Association (ASHA). Within the context of each of these programs, undergraduate and graduate level students must earn a minimum of 400 hours of supervised clinical practicum across at least three different clinical settings. This means that the student must gain experience in university clinics, hospitals, community clinics, schools, skilled nursing facilities, and rehabilitation facilities with a wide diversity of clients representing many different types of communication disorders. Across all of these practicum settings and types of clients, the student in training is expected to participate in a variety of professional communications, both verbal and written.

CLINICAL SETTINGS

As stated earlier, students are expected to participate in practicum experiences across a variety of work settings before they earn their graduate degree. The three most common types of clinical environments that students will encounter are university clinics, medical settings (e.g., hospitals, rehabilitation centers, nursing homes), and public schools. When students are initially placed in each of these three types of settings, they instantly notice that there are significant differences among the environments in terms of clients, the pace of assessment/treatment, and paperwork requirements. We would like to take some time now to clarify a couple of misconceptions students often have about how these settings relate to one another. First, it is important to realize that each setting is unique and there is no way that a particular type of facility can substitute for a different type of operation. For example, the university setting is typically a community clinic and cannot operate as a school or hospital. There is no way we can place beds in a university clinic or do video studies of swallowing. Likewise, we cannot use the university to act as an elementary school for large groups of children with communication disorders. University clinic training acts as a sheltered environment for initial clinical experiences and is not meant to substitute for or emulate medical or educational placements. In fact, some training programs do not even

have an on-campus clinic and students will have to get all of their training off-site.

As mentioned above, students are sent to off-campus sites to gain unique clinical experiences that are not available in a university clinic. Sometimes students will complain that they have not been given practicum experience in dealing with swallowing disorders at the university clinic and have engaged only in classroom study of the issues. When they go to a hospital, they have their first hands-on experience with dysphagia. Of course, that is exactly why they were sent to the medical placement: to obtain experience that is not available in the university clinic. That is a good thing, not a deficiency in the university training program. Second, no one type of setting is superior to another. The sites are merely different. Students sometimes come back to the university after an off-campus medical placement and tell us that the experiences they had in the training program do not reflect the "real world" of the hospital or rehabilitation center. Of course, these medical placements do not reflect the real world of the public schools either, and vice versa. Students often forget that the university training program has a goal of exposing them to the real world, and this is accomplished through off-campus placements and internship experiences. Thus, it is simply not accurate to say that the university does not reflect real world practices; it systematically provides students with exposure to such settings through practicum experiences. University training programs are neither better nor worse than other placements; they are just different. At the university we try to present all of the relevant information and we may not necessarily tailor it to a particular work setting. That part is done by the supervising professionals who are working in medical settings and school systems. There may be many scientifically supported approaches to assessment and treatment that are "ideal," and these may have to be modified to be appropriate in medical or school settings. Thus, students should not think of one setting as being wrong when there are simply different ways of approaching clinical work in each one.

Some of the differences among settings flow from regulatory agencies (e.g., ASHA, Medicare, private insurance, Department of Education, etc.) and others stem from the "culture" of each work envi-

Table 2–1. Practicum Setting Comparison Chart: Regulatory Control

	University	*Medical*	*School*
ASHA Regulations	• Heavily regulated by ASHA • Must train knowledges and skills • Accreditation requirements • Professional practice standards	• Not regulated by ASHA • Only professional practice standards and code of ethics apply	• Not regulated by ASHA
Federal Medicare Regulations	• No Medicare regulations unless clinic is a Medicare provider	• Heavily regulated by Medicare for adult clients	• Not regulated by Medicare
Federal Medicaid Regulations	• No Medicaid regulations unless clinic is a Medicaid provider	• Heavily regulated by Medicaid for child clients	• Not all systems regulated by Medicaid unless they bill Medicaid
Federal Education Regulations	• No federal education regulations	• No federal education regulations	• Heavily regulated by federal education department
State Education Regulations	• No state education regulations	• No state education regulations	• Heavily regulated by state education department
Federal Hospital Regulations	• No federal hospital regulations	• Heavily regulated by national guidelines	• No federal hospital regulations
State Hospital Regulations	• No state hospital regulations	• Heavily regulated by state guidelines	• No state hospital regulations
Third-Party Payer Influence (e.g., insurance companies)	• Some clients use third-party payers • Some insurance carriers limit the amount and type of assessment/treatment paid for	• Insurance companies regulate number and length of sessions paid for • Insurance companies regulate types of treatment reimbursed • Assessment and treatment are often driven by administrative regulations for billable hours	• No third-party payers

ronment. Table 2–1 shows the differences in regulatory agencies that dictate how each setting operates. University training programs are run a particular way because ASHA accreditation hangs in the balance. Medical settings are hamstrung by federal and state regulations, Medicare/Medicaid regulations, and insurance companies. Educational settings have a myriad of federal and state regulations to abide by

in conducting their business. Table 2–2 depicts some of the differences in clinical operation in terms of caseload, supervision, and reporting. Just considering these primal differences among work settings should help you to understand why your practicum experiences will change dramatically depending on where you are assigned. We elaborate on each work setting in the following sections.

Table 2–2. Practicum Setting Comparison Chart: Clinical Operation

	University	*Medical*	*School*
Caseload Issues	• Total control of caseload • Caseload determined by number of students and faculty and availability of clinical facilities	• Typically large caseloads • Little control of caseload	• Typically large caseloads • Little control of caseload • Legal mandates to provide free services to all qualified children
Pressure to Earn Income for Clinic	• Clinic income not usually the basis for faculty salaries • Often have sliding fee scale where patients pay according to income level and family size	• Pressure to generate billable hours • Income may be used to pay salaries and benefits	• Treatment does not produce income because it is free
Time Limitations on Clinical Work	• No time limitations on length of evaluations or treatment sessions	• Limitation on amount of time that can be billed to Medicare or third-party payers	• Limitation on assessment and treatment time imposed by large caseloads and local regulations
Reports and Paperwork	• Reports are typically designed to teach clinicians to provide complete, accurate information • Reports may be lengthy with room for narrative explanations of case history information and interpretation • Greatest opportunity for lengthy reports	• Reports are extremely brief and may be limited to checklists with few opportunities for narrative • Reports may be in electronic format in a paperless environment • Least opportunity for lengthy reports	• Reports may include narratives, test scores or, depending on the school system, a form with check boxes. • Treatment reports are often the IEP • Moderate opportunity for lengthy reports

The University Setting

Figure 2–1 shows a university setting, depicted as a series of "ivory towers" surrounded by several pictures. We have the ubiquitous professor lecturing to a class and another picture of a classroom using multimedia. Another picture shows a student dragging himself to the classroom with questionable motivation. The picture of the hand helping the person up the stairway symbolizes the sheltered environment of the training program where academic and clinical faculty are there to assist you if you have difficulty. Books, of course, are part of the deal in a training program, and we are aware that your tendency will be to sell them, but try to resist it so you won't have

to buy them all back for your professional library. Graduation and receiving your diploma are obviously the main goals; you want to be a certified speech-language pathologist who graduated with a master's degree from an accredited program. Finally, the stadium represents some of the extracurricular activities that are part of college life. Enjoy your experience as a student, because as you reach the end of your training program, it begins to approximate the feeling of a "real job." In our program, for example, students finish their master's training with a full-time internship in some sort of medical or educational facility where they are working from 8:00 to 5:00 every day. Their major comment is usually that they are tired at the end of the day and are thankful they do not have to study for classes and take examinations. These

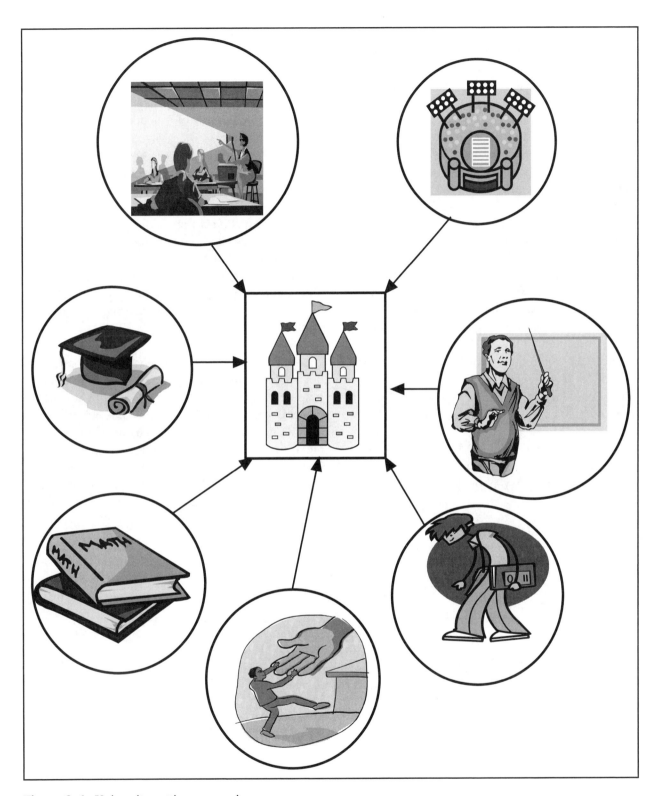

Figure 2–1. University settings are unique.

same students will graduate, do their clinical fellowship (CF), and then they will no longer be students at all, but professionals with jobs, mortgages, and car payments. And take our word for it, you will long for those days when you were a student with less responsibility and much more free time. It's all part of growing up. The pictures we selected in Figure 2–1 are certainly not representative of all the experiences you might have had at the university; they were selected to portray the ambiance of your time in college. You will see when we begin to discuss other practicum settings that the orbit of pictures circling the hospital and school building are quite different indeed. This is because each setting has its own culture, atmosphere, and mood.

University training programs are largely designed to produce competent clinicians who are eligible for certification. Much of what goes on in the university training program is dictated by ASHA regulations and accreditation requirements. Figure 2–2 illustrates the flow of experiences in a university training program. Following are just some of the specific objectives of a university training program:

■ Teaching a specific knowledge base in normal processes of communication (speech science, anatomy, physiology, phonetics, language acquisition).

■ Teaching a specific knowledge base in disorders of communication involving phonology, language, voice, fluency, and swallowing. This knowledge base must transcend specific settings and represent the most current information and ideal standards of practice with particular disorders.

■ Providing a scientific basis or rationale for assessment and treatment of communication disorders.

■ Providing a sheltered environment for initial forays into clinical practice.

■ Providing students constructive feedback on developing clinical skills.

■ Coordinating additional practicum experiences in unique settings for experiences that are not available in the university speech and hearing clinic.

University clinics typically have limited caseloads due to the regulations on supervision of students in training. Students must be supervised by a certified professional at least 25% of the time for treatment and 50% of the time for assessment. These requirements make it difficult for a university clinic to amass several hundred clients, due to the limitations of student clinicians and the constraint of having enough clinical supervisors. As a result, the caseloads in

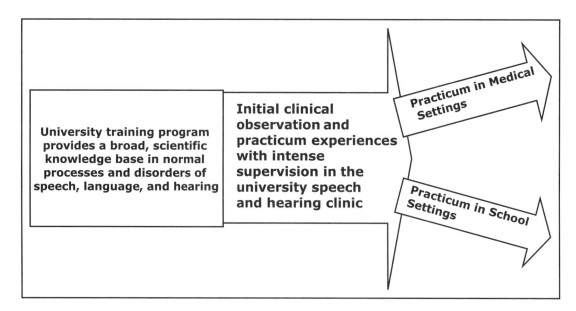

Figure 2–2. Progression of clinical training involving three settings.

university clinics are small enough that clients can be offered assessment and treatment sessions that are longer than in other settings. For instance, clients might be seen for 1-hour sessions of therapy or have a 2-hour evaluation session. Longer sessions are desirable in the university setting because students must gain experience administering a variety of assessment and treatment techniques so they can demonstrate the knowledge and skills required for certification by ASHA. Think of how students and supervisors schedule time to plan for cases and engage in supervisory conferences to talk not only about the client's progress, but your developing skills as a clinician. This is a luxury that the university setting has, but other settings may not due to large caseloads or restrictions of regulatory agencies and insurance companies that will only pay for limited treatment sessions. Most university clinics have no fee for services or offer reduced fees for assessment and treatment. This also may not be seen in many other settings (private practice, hospital, etc.).

It is unique in the university setting that you will typically have little face-to-face communication with teachers, physicians, and other therapists who are also involved in the care of your client. In the public school or medical setting, it is not uncommon to spend a significant part of your day corresponding with other professionals involved in the care of your client as they are on site. Therefore, when treating clients at the university clinic, it will take some effort on your part to find an effective way of communicating with your client's teacher or other therapists to be on the same page.

Another limitation of the university clinic is that this environment cannot recreate the ambience of a hospital or school system. It is difficult to prepare students in university clinics to deal with scenarios involving clients being taken from classrooms for therapy or adult patients who must travel by wheelchair from physical therapy to speech. With regard to report writing, most universities take the view that students in training should produce reports with the most complete data and narrative sections to illustrate the most that can be done with professional writing. At some point in your career, you may be asked to produce a formal report that will be used in a legal case or to establish eligibility for specific services on behalf of a client. In these cases, a simple checklist would not be the most appropriate type of report. There may be a need for explanation of the rationale for treatment and elucidation of how and why treatment targets have changed over time. Thus, university clinics are relatively sheltered environments in which students can be assigned limited numbers of clients and focus intently on the details of assessment, treatment planning, and the "long version" of clinical reporting. ASHA says that a student's initial practicum experiences should be in such a sheltered environment where time can be taken to learn some basics of clinical work prior to going to off-campus settings.

Easing the Transition into Clinical Practicum in the University Clinical Setting

As we said in Chapter 1, professionalism is all about communication. It is through communication that you project yourself as a professional whether it is verbally or in writing. It is important that you are proactive in approaching your clinical practicum and do some planning and preparation for the experience. If you are proactive, some of the fear of the unknown will be lessened and you will gain a certain amount of control over events. In some university clinics, you will have just completed undergraduate classes in the normal processes of speech, hearing, and language and some of the disorders courses when you will have the opportunity to engage in clinical practicum. First, you will have the chance to observe assessment and treatment, and then you will be assigned a client or two of your own for which you take primary responsibility. Some of you might be in a training program that reserves all the cases for the graduate students. In that case, you can use our advice when you start clinical practicum on the graduate level. In most cases, however, undergraduate students have some opportunity to take responsibility for a case, typically in the areas of language or phonology. The case is usually a child, which limits your practicum experience to a specific group of clients. Assuming that you do engage in clinical practicum as an undergraduate, you will feel a distinct difference as you go from a student who takes classes to one who interacts with clients. You go from reading, listening to lectures, studying, and taking tests to planning, executing, and reporting clinical activities. Plus, there is a large increase in the expectation that you will act and communicate professionally. It is quite a jump from being a fairly anonymous student in a class of 30 to being on the spot as a clinical performer. So what advice can we give you to help ease the transition into clinical practicum and make it appear that your professionalism quotient is fairly high? We have some general suggestions:

1. **Look the part:** When you meet with your clinical practicum supervisor for the first time, make sure that you try to appear professional. You must remember that in many cases, your practicum supervisor may have never met you before, and if there was a prior meeting, it was probably in a classroom setting. In some instances, you may never have even had a conversation with one another. So it does not hurt to dress for success and come to your first meeting with a shiny new notebook in which to jot down important information. Remember that professionalism is communicated by your appearance, your demeanor, and the language you use.

2. **Be punctual:** When you have your first meeting, make certain that you are on time. It is extremely important once you begin clinical practicum to make sure you are on time for your scheduled cases; your ability to be on time for a supervisory conference may be seen as a bellwether of your clinical responsibility to clients.

3. **Be prepared by reviewing your case:** When you go for your first supervisory conference, you no doubt will have been assigned a case with whom you will be working. It is always good form to have *extensively* studied the client's file from beginning to end. Do not just read the last report and omit the historical perspective. Supervisors will often ask beginning students to summarize the case as a way of beginning the first conference. If you are not prepared, you run the risk of being perceived as uninterested and unprofessional. Even if you are not asked to summarize the case, it is good policy to be as familiar with your client as possible. Usually, students tend to use the recommendations that were made in the most recent report as a template for planning their current approach to treatment. Although this is very logical, there is nothing wrong with having questions about the treatment approach that was recommended. If you find inconsistencies in the report, it is good to ask for clarification from the supervisor as to why they exist. For example, if the report is recommending the same goals and procedures used in the past semester, but the data show that the client made minimal progress, it would be logical to ask why you would want to spend the next 15 weeks doing what did not work in the past. You can make suggestions about applying concepts from your classroom work to the case as well. At the very least, you should ask questions about how a procedure was actually done in treatment sessions. It is almost impossible to recreate treatment tasks in a clinical report in sufficient detail to be replicated by a new clinician. So asking your supervisor, "Can you give me an example of how this task was actually done in a session?" is not inappropriate. If you can communicate that you are prepared for your first conference, your supervisor will tend to perceive you as having a high degree of professionalism.

4. **Be prepared by reviewing class notes:** Because you will be aware of the type of case you have been assigned, you will know the kind of disorder the client exhibits. For instance, if you are assigned a child with a language disorder, you would be wise to review your notes from the courses you took in language acquisition and language disorders. If the client has specific symptoms or is in a particular stage of language development, you should especially refresh your memory regarding course information on this stage. Your supervisor might ask you a question such as, "What is the next thing to develop in a normal child at this stage of language acquisition?" It does nothing for your professional image if you shrug your shoulders and say, "I don't know." After all, you have taken several courses dealing with the topic and your inability to answer the question means that (a) you learned nothing from the course or (b) you did not prepare for the supervisory conference.

Either of those reasons suggests a less than professional attitude.

5. **Be prepared to write things down:** It is important that you show that you are taking responsibility for your client and ownership of the treatment plan. A good way to communicate this to your supervisor is to take notes. We have had some students have a meeting with us to discuss therapy activities only to hurriedly ask us before their session, "What did we say again?" This not only wastes your supervisor's time but results in you not being prepared and perhaps a less than ideal treatment session. It is good practice to avoid this scenario by writing down specifics when you discuss them with your supervisor. Don't take it for granted that you will remember or falsely assume that your supervisor thinks you should not need to take notes. After you have taken the time to be prepared with thoughtful questions regarding treatment history, you should write down the answers so you will have them to go over later. You may think you will remember it all later but it is always good to have the written information, especially when you have multiple clients that you are planning for. You may be worried that it takes extra time to write the information down; however, we can assure you that it shows your supervisor you are prepared and conscientious. It also provides a valuable resource for you to review when planning for treatment sessions.

6. **Talk with other students if possible:** If your client in the university clinic was seen the previous semester by a student who is still around, it is valuable to contact that clinician and chat about the case. You can gain much insight about the client, the treatment activities, the family, behavioral issues, room arrangement, and other information from a previous clinician. You can also get a preview of how the interaction was between the clinician and your new clinical supervisor. Sometimes the student will tell you some things to avoid: "Ms. Smith really hates it when you don't bring data to your conferences." Other advice might be on the positive side of the ledger: "She lets you use some of the therapy materials from her office." Get as much

information as possible about your client, from any sources available to you.

7. **Use professional language:** As much as possible, try to use appropriate terminology when talking to your supervisor. For example, do not call phonemes "speech sounds" when you know the appropriate term.

8. **Define your responsibilities:** During the first conference make certain that you know what you are expected to do each week and throughout the semester. It goes without saying that you will be expected to be present for your therapy sessions. There are other meetings and responsibilities, however, that may not be as clear to you initially. For instance, you will probably have to schedule a supervisory conference on a weekly basis to discuss your case and your developing clinical skills. If the meeting time is ongoing from week to week, block it out on your calendar. Make sure you know what is to be done during these conferences. For example, the supervisor may want you to bring treatment data on the client's goals to each meeting. If you do not bring it, there is little to talk about in the meeting and you are perceived as not meeting one of your professional obligations. Are you expected to generate a therapy plan each week? Are you expected to place a case summary devoid of identifying information in the observation room to assist observers? Do you have to write progress notes each week? Where are they and what is the format? Are you expected to transcribe language samples periodically to monitor progress? Is there a midterm progress report due on a particular date? When does treatment end and when is the final report due to the supervisor? What is your role in contacting other professionals working with your case (e.g., school system, psychologist) to coordinate programs or check on generalization? What is expected of you regarding parent counseling or devising a home program to assist in generalization? All of these questions are important for you to ask or clarify if they are not already addressed by your clinical supervisor. They show that you are interested in the case and professional in your involvement. As

clinical supervisors, we can tell you that we welcome as many questions as it takes for you to completely understand your responsibilities.

9. **Determine how you will be evaluated:** The interaction between you and your clinical supervisor has two major goals. First, both you and your supervisor want the client to be given appropriate services and make progress as a result. A second goal that is unique to training programs is that the supervisor wants to see your own clinical behavior change over time. It is important that you ask how and when you will be evaluated and how your grade in clinical practicum will be determined. In most cases, there are evaluation forms that your supervisor will share with you that show the behaviors and attributes she uses in grading your clinical competence. Sometimes supervisors leave notes after every session to provide feedback to students. Some programs evaluate students midway through the semester and again at the end. However your supervisor provides feedback, it is critical that you get it often and early enough in the semester to make changes in your behavior. If you are not getting enough feedback, do not be shy about asking for it.

10. **Other expectations:** Be certain to clarify any expectations that go beyond the therapy session itself. For example, be familiar with clinic guidelines about infection control, disinfecting toys/ materials, checking out of materials/tests, and returning the treatment room to its original condition for the next clinician. Also make sure you are aware of periodic meetings or staffings that you are expected to attend.

The Medical Setting

Figure 2–3 attempts to illustrate the mood of the medical setting. Note that it is considerably different from the university environment. Professionals wear specific clothing, in most cases "scrubs," which make everyone from a skilled surgeon to the maintenance personnel look like doctors. Patients, depending on their units, may be wearing hospital gowns or street clothes. Some patients are in bed and others travel by a variety of different conveyances such as wheelchairs, walkers, and canes. Some patients are hooked up to equipment such as IV stands or oxygen tanks. There is an obvious emphasis on infection control as evidenced by a smell of disinfectant and copious boxes of latex gloves. All of a sudden, you are working with other professionals from physical therapy (PT), occupational therapy (OT), respiratory therapy (RT), and nursing. You get the distinct feeling that you are not in Kansas anymore. In medical settings such as hospitals, rehabilitation centers, and skilled nursing facilities, there is a whole new set of regulatory influences on clinical practice. Whereas ASHA was the 800-pound gorilla in the university setting, medical environments are under no regulatory constraints from this organization. As indicated in Table 2–1, medical settings are mostly regulated by federal and state hospital guidelines, Medicare, Medicaid, and third-party payers such as insurance companies. These influences will have a direct impact on how long you can see your patient, the goals you address, and paperwork associated with medical settings.

With regard to your training, medical settings have the following goals:

- Exposing students to varied caseloads of medically based communication disorders in children and adults.
- Exposing students to the physical facilities common for hospitals, rehabilitation centers, and skilled nursing residences.
- Exposing students to allied professionals (e.g., nurses, physical therapists, occupational therapists, physicians, radiologists) typically encountered in medical settings.
- Exposing students to the unique culture of medical settings with its attendant terminologies, equipment, and paperwork requirements.

When we refer to medical settings in this book, we are including acute care hospitals, inpatient rehabilitation facilities (IRF), and skilled nursing facilities (SNF). While these settings have some overlap, they are each unique and patients' experiences vary according to their diagnoses and payment source. The length of stay (LOS) may average several days in an acute care setting to several weeks in an inpatient rehabilitation facility. Although skilled nursing facilities have some beds designated "rehab" beds in

Figure 2–3. Medical settings are unique.

which patients stay for a period of time before discharging home or elsewhere, patients often remain until the end of their life. Admission criteria to IRFs and SNFs varies again according to patient status and their payment source. Unlike in the university clinic where patients can attend therapy for as long as they wish, therapy is limited to a specific number of sessions or length of time.

When students go to a medical setting for the first time they are usually in a state of shock. First, the pace is considerably faster in medical settings because there are many more clients who are seen for shorter sessions as compared to the university clinic. In the hospital or rehabilitation environment, everyone is using terminologies that are unique to the medical setting, and students new to this environment are often intimidated by this unique language. Also, the student is interacting with other professionals in physical therapy, occupational therapy, respiratory therapy, and nursing, all of whom have their own jargon you have to learn and understand. Patients will be arriving in wheelchairs or using walkers or tripod canes. The patients may have just been to physical or occupational therapy and now must battle fatigue to participate in language treatment. Often, the clients the student dealt with in the university clinic were children with language and phonological disorders, and now the patients are adults who have neurogenically based communication problems or dysphagia. There will probably be less time spent in supervisory conferences as compared to the university. In some cases, a facility will have a standard protocol for dealing with treatment or assessment plans, and very little actual planning will be required of the student beyond how to implement the program. In some settings there may be a standard set of treatment materials in the form of a workbook that the student and client will use.

One of the biggest changes students see in medical settings is the different way of reporting assessment and treatment activity. The most noticeable difference is the brevity of reporting in medical settings. Students will do assessments in 30 minutes, and the "report" may only be a form that includes boxes to check with a few lines available for a narrative sentence or two. In IRFs, a patient's functional independence measure (FIM) score will mean more to the third-party payers than will your narrative sentences. A patient's length of stay in the facility is dependent upon the numbers they are assigned upon admission. The patient's chart is a central point of communication in medical settings and the patient's status and progress must be summarized for other professionals to read. This is quite different from the lengthy narrative reports the student has written in university clinics. The chart in the medical setting allows each of the professionals involved in the patient's care to document their interactions with the patient. Charting in these locations can be fairly short and includes pertinent information only. The patient's known case history information, plan of care, physician's orders, nurses' notes, therapist notes, and notes regarding medical exams/procedures are all included in the chart. The chart is kept in a central location, usually the nurses' station, to allow all professionals equal access. While you should omit flowery and verbose descriptions while making chart notes, you should remember the common saying "If it's not written in the chart, it didn't happen." Therefore, if you don't document that you educated a patient regarding their safe swallow strategies and they say you didn't, you are held accountable for not providing them with the information.

Students often complain that one of the most difficult things about professional reporting in the medical setting is learning how to communicate clinical results in a brief and economical format. What took an entire paragraph in a university report might only be communicated in a sentence or phrase in a patient's chart. It is not unusual for students who have completed a rotation in a medical setting to come strutting back into the university clinic in their scrubs and suggest that all of the time and detail spent on clinical reports in the training program were overkill and not reflective of the real world. It is important to remember, however, that before one can scale down information for a medical chart, she has to know what she is talking about. One cannot fully appreciate the elegance of a well-crafted, parsimonious phrase unless she understands exactly how the economical version really does reflect the reality of the patient's progress. We should always remember that checking boxes on an assessment form is often done at the expense of distorting the view of the patient.

Easing the Transition to Medical Practicum Settings

It is important to realize that when you arrive at a new practicum setting, you are not only representing yourself as a burgeoning professional, but you are also acting as a representative of your training program. Thus, it is critical that you think very carefully about the first impression you give to the professionals in your new practicum setting. Remember, the SLPs working in a hospital, rehabilitation center, or nursing facility are true professionals who have their own reputations to consider, as well as the reputation of their unit in the medical setting. Medical settings are divided into a host of different departments such as radiology, psychology, SLP, physical therapy, occupational therapy, and so on. Each unit has its departmental reputation to protect, and each professional working in the department is ultimately responsible for the actions of practicum students they supervise. If you create difficulties or act unprofessionally, it reflects not only on your immediate supervisor, but on that person's department and the university training program as well. So, like it or not, the pressure is on and the ball is in your court. You will remember that we promised to give you some good advice to ease the transition into different practicum settings, so in the next few sections, help is on the way.

We indicated earlier in the present chapter that a major purpose of this text is to assist students in developing professional attitudes and behaviors. One way of doing that is to think *proactively* as you move through your clinical practicum. We have tried to illustrate that one stumbling block in your practicum experience might be the differences you will encounter in the various types of work settings to which you are assigned. Knowing that you will have to make some adjustments in how you act and perform various tasks should be a first step to regaining control. It is important that you do some thinking and planning before you arrive at a strange practicum site. Be prepared to present yourself as a professional in training who has certain competencies but has come to the medical setting to learn more. Obviously, you are not coming to the hospital setting because you are a seasoned veteran who knows what to do. You have some knowledge from classes, and you might have even worked with some clients in the university clinic who have medically related communication disorders. On the other hand, this may be your first experience with medical SLP. Whatever your situation, you can still make a good first impression on your new practicum supervisor(s). It is critical, however, that you not merely waltz into the hospital and say, "I'm here!" Adequate preparation on your part will make all the difference when meeting your supervisors for the first time. Following are some areas you might consider in planning your first visit to a new practicum site:

1. **Prepracticum visit:** When possible, we recommend that instead of just showing up on your first day of scheduled practicum, you meet with your supervisor ahead of time. We understand that this may not always be feasible; however, it shows that you are interested, serious-minded, and professional. At times, the medical facility may request this meeting before you do to discuss their policies, but regardless of who makes the appointment, it is a good tactic to make a prepracticum visit. Typically, you will be assigned to one supervisor but you would be prudent to ask at your meeting if you will be rotating among several supervisors or shadowing the same one throughout your practicum.

2. **Orientation:** During your prepracticum visit you should ask about any orientation that will be provided by the facility for new practicum students. Again, your new supervisor may be planning to introduce this topic, but if she does not, you should ask. If the supervisor begins by telling you about a mandatory orientation meeting, you can say, "Good. That was one of the things I was going to ask about, and I'm so glad that an orientation is available." Orientations are frequently required before your internship for the purpose of educating you about privacy laws and policies, infection control and specific facility protocols.

3. **Being honest about your training:** Although practicum supervisors may see many students from university training programs, the students may have different levels of experience in medical SLP. It is important that you are honest about

your coursework and practicum experiences at the university. If you have obvious gaps in your knowledge and experience, it is fine to tell your new supervisor what you feel comfortable with and in which areas you still have a lot to learn. It is especially important to communicate your interest in learning new things and that you appreciate the opportunity to learn as much as possible during your practicum experience. Supervisors do not expect you to "know it all," just be willing to try and receptive to instruction and suggestions.

4. **Learn names and the organizational structure:** Obviously, it is important for you to write down the names of any people you will be interacting with on a daily basis in the practicum placement. Do not be afraid to jot down those names because it is not unusual for you to meet many people during a visit including the SLP staff, people from other disciplines (physical therapy, occupational therapy, physicians, nurses), patients, hospital administrators, secretarial staff, and other practicum students. It makes a good impression when you return if you can remember the names of people you met during your visit. Perhaps even more important than remembering names is figuring out the organizational structure of the facility in which you will be working. Like any organization, medical facilities have a power structure that is important to learn if you are going to be working there. For example, the SLP unit may be comprised of three SLPs, one of whom has administrative responsibility over the department. The speech-pathology unit may be part of a larger department that includes physical therapy, occupational therapy, respiratory therapy, and some other types of allied health professions. There is an administrator who oversees all of these different types of therapy and the SLP coordinator has to answer to this person. Our point here is that it is important for you to see where you are in the organizational arrangement of your medical facility and who is in charge at various levels. You never know when you will need to work with other departments and general offices such as risk management, security, or administrative offices. Your supervisor will tell you who is most

important for you to know about while you are completing your practicum experience.

5. **Handouts:** It is appropriate for you to ask about the availability of any orientation handouts or brochures that cover policies and procedures of the facility in general and the SLP section in particular. Many practicum sites have informative manuals they have constructed just for practicum students to orient them to the setting. It is almost impossible for you to write down everything you are told in a prepracticum visit, so asking for a handout shows that you are interested in and serious about adhering to the rules and guidelines of the facility.

6. **Your schedule:** It is important to ask specific questions about your schedule such as when to arrive each day, where to report when you arrive, where to park, and when to leave. You cannot be punctual if you do not know your schedule. This would be a good time to have your supervisor describe a typical day you might experience, from start to finish. You should also ask about special events that will concern you (e.g., accreditation visits, hospital or department meetings). Please remember that flexibility is key, especially in medical settings where you are treating sick people. It is likely that some days you may have to stay longer than your scheduled time to finish your work for the day. In most cases, your schedule will mirror that of your assigned supervisor, so if he or she is staying late, you will be expected to as well, and with a smile on your face!

7. **Responsibilities:** This is also a good time to ask about your responsibilities as a practicum student and how they might change as you gain more experience. You should ask about supervision in terms of how frequently it is provided and the opportunities for supervisory conferences regarding your caseload. Asking about the evaluation forms that will be used to grade your clinical work would also be appropriate at this time. It is possible that in some settings you will not see patients alone in the beginning. You may be observing or working with the facility SLP jointly at first. The supervisor can tell you how they work with practicum students, and you should be interested in this. It would be

good to know that during a 15-week practicum experience, greater responsibility will gradually be shifted to you as you progress in the training.

8. **The facilities:** Ask for a tour of the facilities and where you will be seeing patients for assessment and treatment. Will you go to a dedicated room? Will you see some patients in their hospital room? Will you be working with groups? Where will group therapy be held?

9. **Transport:** Medical facilities have various regulations about transporting patients. Some patients in wheelchairs are often transported from one therapy to another by aides and sometimes by the person who just finished treating them (such as physical therapy). The point here is that you should be aware of what the conventions are in the facility and how patients get from one place to another. Also, be aware that, while it may not be your job to transport a patient to therapy, you may be required to do this in the event that other personnel are busy. A major issue involves transferring patients from beds to wheelchairs, or vice versa. You should not do this without specific training because of possible injury to the patient or yourself. Find out the procedures that are used in your facility before you start working with patients, or else you could make a big mistake.

10. **Paperwork:** Because you will be required to produce many reports, notes, and other forms of paperwork, it is only logical that you should have the opportunity to look at examples of such output. In some cases, your supervisor will give you examples with identifying information deleted to protect confidentiality. In other cases, you may be given an opportunity to study patient charts in the office. Whatever the case, it is good to familiarize yourself with the types of paperwork you will be asked to generate so that you can come closer to hitting the mark the first try.

11. **Confidentiality:** Ask about how patient confidentiality is handled at the facility. How is paperwork stored and secured? Are there secure computers available on which to do your reports? What disposal methods (shredding, erasing) are available for paperwork, electronic media, and audio/video tapes, and how is disposal accomplished?

The School Setting

In Figure 2–4 we try to capture some of the ambiance of the school setting. First of all, there are many children as opposed to the adults in medical placements. The professionals you deal with are regular education teachers, learning disabilities (LD) teachers, special educators, psychologists, special education coordinators, school administrators, and various support personnel. Children attend classes that focus on literacy, content areas of math, science, history, and social studies, and physical education. The classroom is an important milieu and you hear bells signaling the transition of one class to another or recess or lunchtime. Placement in a school setting also has unique goals in your clinical training. Just as the university clinic and medical setting offer a special dimension to your education, school systems provide yet another facet to your developing skills. Some of the following are goals of the school setting related to your training:

■ Exposing students to the varied caseload of the public schools ranging from preschool to adolescence. These caseloads can range from relatively simple disorders of articulation and language to very complex problems involving swallowing, augmentative communication, head injury, vocal disorders, and stuttering.

■ Exposing students to the physical facilities typically seen in school settings from preschool programs to secondary schools.

■ Exposing students to allied professionals (e.g., teachers, special educators, psychologists, aides, administrators) typically encountered in the school setting.

■ Exposing students to the culture of the educational setting with its attendant terminology, equipment, and paperwork requirements.

One thing that is immediately noticeable is that children are being seen for treatment in small groups, as well as individually. The school SLP may also do therapy within the classroom context and incorporate curriculum materials into treatment activities. As indicated in Table 1–1, schools are primarily

Figure 2–4. School settings are unique.

regulated by federal and state departments of education. There are a series of laws that dictate how business is conducted in school systems ranging from the Individuals with Disabilities Education Act (IDEA) and No Child Left Behind (depending on your state's laws) to Section 504 of the Rehabilitation Act and the Americans with Disabilities Act (ADA). These guidelines will be discussed in later chapters; however, they are mentioned here to illustrate that schools are controlled by a myriad of legal guidelines coming from the state and federal government. Caseloads in the schools are typically high, which makes group therapy a more efficient way of providing services. School systems have very systematic procedures, just as medical facilities do for identifying clients and providing treatment. Specific forms, such as the *Individualized Education Program* (IEP), are standard fare in school systems, and we will talk more about these in a later chapter. Services are provided free of charge, which is a major difference from most other settings. Unfortunately, although the law says that every student should be provided adequate treatment, some school systems may be underfunded and not have enough personnel or facilities to service every child ideally. Other systems have state-of-the-art facilities, a full complement of highly qualified faculty, and small caseloads. Just as hospital settings vary in size, quality, and in terms of personnel, school systems do as well. Remember that school systems must service children from age 3 to 21, and many districts are providing assessment and treatment from birth onward. School systems use a variety of models to provide services including direct therapy, group therapy, consultative, center-based, and home-based programs. Thus, your practicum experience in the school environment can be quite varied. In the past, the stereotype of a school system was that the caseload was largely made up of language and articulation cases. Today, schools represent one of the most diverse caseload environments available in clinical practice. It is not unusual to see children with head injury, unique syndromes, stuttering, voice disorders, cerebral palsy, autism, swallowing problems, and hearing impairments. There are children in the regular classroom who are on ventilators and who must use an augmentative communication device. Many of the children have been diagnosed with learning disabilities, attention defi-

cit disorder, psychological difficulties, and behavior problems. Thus, the school environment is different from medical or university settings and this uniqueness is seen in assessment, treatment, reporting, and every other aspect of clinical work.

Easing the Transition to School Practicum Settings

Just as we urged you to be proactive in transitioning into your first practicum case in the university clinic and your introduction to a medical setting, we again suggest planning for your first visit to a school placement. Many of the principles we suggested for the other two settings also apply to practicum in the schools and we do not provide as much detail here:

1. **Prepracticum visit:** As in the medical setting, we recommend that you visit the school setting prior to your first day of practicum so that you can ask questions and receive instructions from your supervisor.
2. **Orientation:** In some school systems there will be an orientation provided for new practicum students. Be sure to ask about this and attend if it is offered.
3. **Be honest about your training:** In the school system you have a higher likelihood of working with children who have language and phonological disorders. This, in some ways, might be similar to your experience at the university clinic. You will have a larger comfort zone with these clients than you will have with medically oriented disorders in a hospital setting. Thus, you should feel a bit more comfortable in the school setting. Share with your practicum supervisor the types of experiences you have had in the university clinic.
4. **Learn names and the organizational structure:** As in the medical setting, there will be many names for you to learn in the school placement: the SLP(s), school nurse, school psychologist, many regular classroom teachers, special education teachers, learning disabilities specialists, reading teachers, school administrators such as principals and assistant principals, a special education coordinator, and the secretarial staff. To compound this, you will often be assigned

to multiple school buildings and so the names increase exponentially. The school organizational structure is both similar to and different from the medical setting. Schools tend to have a superintendent who oversees the entire school system. Each school is run administratively by a principal and assistant principal who control what happens in their building. An SLP is typically under a special education coordinator who might oversee psychology, SLP, learning disabilities, special education, and reading disabilities. Thus, although you might be supervised by an SLP, you both may be ultimately responsible to the special education coordinator. In some large school systems there might actually be an SLP department composed of many SLPs, and one is designated as the head of the department. It just depends on the size of the school system. No matter where you are assigned, it is important to note where you fit into the organizational structure and to whom you are responsible.

5. **Handouts:** If the school system has any handouts on its policies, it is a good idea to obtain these and become familiar with them prior to your practicum. There may also be handouts generated by the SLP department that are designed for practicum students.

6. **Your schedule:** Like any work setting, there will be expectations regarding when you will arrive for work, when you can leave, and where you will go during the work day. School systems often have employees sign in and out of school buildings. You should ask specifically about your typical daily schedule and any special events (e.g., assemblies, staffings, IEP meetings) that you will be expected to attend.

7. **Responsibilities:** As in the medical setting, your supervisor might start you off with limited responsibilities and increase them as you gain more experience. You should ask about your initial responsibilities and how they are likely to change over time. This would be a good time to ask about the caseload you will be working with in terms of types of disorders, severity, and frequency of therapy. You should also ask if you are seeing the children individually, in groups, or in the classroom setting. This allows you to anticipate the types of activities you will need to prepare for treatment.

8. **Facilities:** You will want to know where you will be working with children in the school. Is there a dedicated speech pathology room? Is most of the treatment done in the classroom setting? Are you sharing a room with other professionals?

9. **Transport:** It is important to determine how the children will get to your treatment sessions. Will you go to the classroom and escort them to therapy? Will the children of a certain age be trusted to come to therapy by themselves? Will the teacher remind them?

10. **Paperwork:** The school system has unique paperwork compared to other settings. You will need to become familiar with IEPs and individual family service plans (IFSPs) and many other forms generated by the school system. It would be helpful if you could obtain example copies of such forms with identifying information removed so that you can approximate these models in your initial attempts at generating paperwork. We discuss these in later chapters and have some examples in the appendices.

11. **Confidentiality:** In all settings you will be required to maintain confidentiality about your clients. You should ask about this issue in the school setting and determine how information is safeguarded and disposed of when no longer needed.

This chapter aimed to introduce you to aspects of your upcoming clinical practicum that students rarely contemplate. Most students think of their practicum experience as a unified, seamless progression that is part of their clinical training. They rarely realize that there are unavoidable adjustments and bumps in the road that will make them question their abilities and the wisdom of those who designed their training program. Hopefully, this chapter has demonstrated to you that moving from one practicum site to another invariably means adjusting what you know and learning new approaches to old problems. The inevitability of having to make adjustments to different practicum settings allows you to anticipate these bumps in the road and take proactive steps to make the transition a bit more comfortable. The following chapters are designed to help you plan for different practicum placements and their attendant diverse environments, approaches to clinical work, and demands for professional communication.

3 Ethics, Confidentiality, and Safeguarding Clinical Communications

The field of speech-language pathology (SLP) is as diverse as it is dynamic and serves a large population of clients. This, in turn, makes speech pathology a public service. Those in the field recognize that the well-being of the people we serve comes first. To that end, confidentiality and safeguarding all information regarding our clients and patients are paramount.

Due to modern technology, public as well as private information is more accessible than ever before. As a result, identity theft and fraudulent use of confidential information has become commonplace. The need for guidelines to ensure the confidentiality of patients under any doctor's or specialist's care was not only recognized by the health care providers themselves but also by the federal government.

In 1996, President Bill Clinton signed the Health Information Portability and Accountability Act, or HIPAA, also known as Public Law 104-191. One of the provisions of HIPAA was to establish measures that ensure the security and privacy of health care information maintained by health care providers, both public and private.

How this relates to speech pathology encompasses many things. Private practices, hospitals, rehabilitation facilities, and long-term care facilities have many forms of communication that contain patient information. Most of this information is viewed by a diverse group of people involved in the patient's care. As a result, the speech-language pathologist may discuss patient and client issues with other relevant professionals on a daily basis. Referrals to other agencies may be made, resulting in information being passed via mail or electronically. It is imperative that the patient's information is protected so that abuse of any kind does not occur.

In addition, clients and caregivers have a legal right to read any report containing information about themselves or their family members (Family Educational Rights & Privacy Act of 1974, Public Law 93-380 [FERPA]). To this end, providers of SLP services must be accountable, not only in keeping accurate data regarding progress made in therapy, but in protecting the privacy of the clients they serve. Another fun fact about FERPA is how it impacts students. You would be surprised at how many calls your professors receive from concerned parents who want to know how you are doing in classes. According to the law, we cannot discuss student performance without your expressed permission. So, even though you might not have known about it, your privacy is being protected by the law. We hope, of course, that you are proud of your performance and share it with your parents, but it is your right to keep them in the dark, if you so desire.

ASHA CODE OF ETHICS

As professionals who are governed by a licensing board, we also have an ethical responsibility to our clients and patients. The American Speech-Language-Hearing Association (ASHA) has a code of ethics (ASHA, 2010) just as other professional organizations such as psychology, medicine, nursing, occupational therapy, education, and physical therapy prescribe ethical responsibilities of practitioners. We do not want to turn this chapter into a review of the entire Code of Ethics on issues such as practice, but would like to mention certain ethical proscriptions that deal with professional communication.

Several portions of the ASHA Code of Ethics relate to the notions of professionalism and communication. We quote these directly from the 2010 version of the Code of Ethics, and you should be able to see how they relate to *professionalism* and *communication* (ASHA, 2010):

■ "Individuals shall not reveal, without authorization, any professional or personal information about identified persons served professionally or identified participants involved in research and scholarly activities unless doing so is necessary to protect the welfare of the person or of the community, or is otherwise required by law" (Principle of Ethics I, Rule N).

■ "Individuals shall fully inform the persons they serve of the nature and possible effects of services rendered and products dispensed, and they shall inform participants in research about the possible effects of their participation in research conducted" (Principle of Ethics I, Rule H).

■ "Individuals shall not guarantee the results of any treatment or procedure, directly or by implication; however, they may make a reasonable statement of prognosis" (Principle of Ethics I, Rule J).

■ "Individuals shall not misrepresent their credentials, competence, education, training, experience, or scholarly or research contributions" (Principle of Ethics III, Rule A).

■ "Individuals shall not misrepresent research, diagnostic information, services rendered, results of services rendered, products dispensed or the effects of products dispensed" (Principle of Ethics III, Rule D).

■ "Individuals' statements to the public shall provide accurate information about the nature and management of communication disorders, about the professions, about professional services, about products for sale, and about research and scholarly activities" (Principle of Ethics III, Rule F).

■ "Individuals' statements to the public when advertising, announcing, and marketing their professional services; reporting research results; and promoting products shall adhere to professional standards and shall not contain misrepresentations" (Principle of Ethics III, Rule G).

■ "Individuals shall not engage in dishonesty, fraud, deceit, or misrepresentation" (Principle of Ethics IV, Rule C).

■ "Individuals' statements to colleagues about professional services, research results, and products shall adhere to prevailing professional standards and shall contain no misrepresentations" (Principle of Ethics IV, Rule I).

The word *professional* appears in almost all of these ethical guidelines. Note also that almost all of them also include the notion of "communication" either explicitly or implicitly. Many of the statements have a great deal to do with the idea that an SLP is expected to communicate with colleagues and patients accurately, in a professional manner, without misrepresenting his clinical practice. Even in our advertising we must meet "professional standards" and not place an advertisement as if we were selling used automobiles. It is no coincidence that announcements and advertising from many different professions (e.g., physicians, dentists, psychologists) all look similar. Thus, we hope you can see that our Code of Ethics places a great deal of emphasis on professional communication. In the next few sections we will zero in on the notion of confidentiality in both written and verbal professional communication across work settings.

THE UNIVERSITY SPEECH AND HEARING CLINIC

The university speech and hearing clinic will be your first foray into dealing with confidential clinical information and acting with a degree of professionalism. If you are not already aware of it, all of our clients deserve the right to privacy in seeking clinical services. Some of them take it quite seriously. We have worked with adult clients who have specifically requested that they not be observed by students in our training program. Although we would like to give students the opportunity to view all treatment sessions, we have to respect the rights of our clients to their privacy. Some clients request privacy only in the beginning of treatment, and then as they gain expertise in communication they are proud of their accomplishments and welcome observers.

George Adams was a retired history professor whose progressive Parkinson's disease essentially put a stop to his teaching career. He had an extremely tremulous voice and made uncontrolled upper body movements even sitting in a chair. Because Dr. Adams had taught at the university for 40 years, he came to the speech and hearing clinic for services. Because he had only retired a year ago he was concerned that some of his former students would still be around to see the ravages of Parkinson's disease on his appearance and communication. He specifically requested that no students be allowed to observe his treatment sessions.

Michael (Michelle) Genrette had made a most drastic decision. He had decided to begin the process of sexual reassignment and become a woman. This very personal decision was not made lightly and Mr. Genrette had undergone extensive counseling from physicians and psychologists. As part of his transition from male to female he had to learn new vocal production patterns, nonverbal communication, and language structures common to women. Mr. Genrette was a faculty member at the university, and he had not yet shared his decision with coworkers or even some of his family members. Thus, it was important for the speech and hearing clinic staff to maintain confidentiality and not talk openly about this case. Mr. Genrette also requested that no one observe his treatment sessions.

The university training program is a veritable minefield of confidentiality issues. First, we generate reams of paperwork related to assessment, treatment, and student training. Second, much of this paperwork is handled on a daily basis by students who have never been responsible for protecting the personal privacy of clients. In the university speech clinic, sources of personal information include, but are not limited to:

- Daily notes and treatment plans
- Formal treatment reports
- Formal diagnostic reports
- Information on flash drives
- Electronic transmissions (faxes, e-mails, billing)
- Authorization forms signed by clients
- Therapy schedules
- Verbal discussions
- Video/audio recordings

Each of these is discussed in more detail below.

Treatment Plans and Progress Notes

The treatment plan and progress note are a vital part of the SLP's daily routine in a university clinic. The treatment plan details the clinician's specific plan for the session, which may include the goals to be targeted and the procedures, cues and reinforcement that will be implemented. In the university clinic, the student writes a treatment plan prior to the session and a progress note after the session. The progress note provides accountability for what takes places in the clinical session through the documentation of data collection, assessment of a client's performance, and plans for future sessions. Both notes may be kept in a client file separate from the permanent record. These files should only be accessible to clinicians and supervisors as part of the safeguarding procedure. The progress note and treatment plan may contain less personal information about the client, as the student may use a client's file number, date of birth, or initials as identifying information. However, if any form is discarded, it should be shredded rather than thrown anyway. No client information should leave the clinic at any point.

Formal Treatment Reports

The formal treatment report includes identifying information, data, and a summary of client performance that usually covers one semester. These reports include a great deal of personal information about a client such as name, date of birth, address, telephone number, referring physician, diagnosis, and so forth. It is important that this information is not handled casually and that the student or students who are working with this client do not leave these reports in public areas where anyone can read this confidential information.

Copy Confusion

Carmen Jones was in a hurry. Her treatment reports on five clients were due to be turned in to her supervisor in less than an hour. She needed to make three copies of each report for distribution to the client folder, parents, and the school system. Carmen found an open Xerox machine at the local copying store and placed each of her five reports in the feeder tray, pressing the appropriate buttons for three copies each. As the copies came out, Carmen paper-clipped them together in a pile and removed the original from the machine. When the last copy was done, she looked at her watch and realized that she only had 10 minutes to get to the clinic. As Carmen grabbed all her copies and rushed out the door, she was oblivious to the fact that the original from the last report she had copied remained in the document feeder. The next person to use that machine would have a golden opportunity to learn about Tyrone Walker, an elementary school student with autism whose mother places a high value on privacy.

Formal Diagnostic Reports

Just as with the formal treatment report, the diagnostic report also contains a great deal of personal information about a client. In fact, the diagnostic report is likely to contain the most personal data of any of our professional communications. By their very nature, diagnostic reports contain a plethora of historical information, not only about the client, but the family as well. So, if a child exhibits behavior problems, such as bed-wetting or thumb sucking, it is all laid out in the case history. If a child has developed disfluencies since his parents' divorce, it is noted in the historical section of the report. Also included in the case history might be test scores from other professionals who have evaluated the client previously. Some of these, such as IQ scores, are noted in the case history and constitute very sensitive information. If a client is being seen by another professional (e.g., psychologist, physician), this is outlined in the case history. The diagnostic report also includes all of the test results of the SLP evaluation including standard scores and percentile ranks of performance on various assessment instruments. Finally, the report will include the evaluator's interpretation of the test results and the formal diagnosis of a disorder. This report may also include recommendations for referrals to other professionals in addition to a diagnosis and prognosis. It is easy to see that no one would want such personal information to be compromised. Our clients assume that any information they divulge will be treated with confidentiality, and a professional should treat this obligation very seriously.

Rainy Day Reporting

Susan Pierce arrived at the university speech and hearing clinic parking lot just in time to grab the last parking space available. It was a rainy Monday morning and she was not looking forward to her back-to-back schedule of supervisory conferences with speech pathology practicum students. Susan had been a clinical supervisor for 5 years and thought she had "seen it all" with regard to student problems. Struggling to open her umbrella and exit her car at the same time, she immediately stepped into a large puddle adjacent to the driver's side door. It was then that she noticed the paper that was pinned squarely in the water beneath her fashionable black high-heeled pump. Through the water she read the smudged yet legible clinic letterhead; and under that was the section called "Identifying Information," which contained the client's name, address, telephone, and other personal information. Further down was a section devoted to case history, which described the devastation in the wake of a major stroke and the effects on the client's job and family. Although the type was a bit smeared, it was easy to read all the sensitive personal information that had been given in confidence to a caring clinician. Literally hundreds of people pass through this parking lot in a day, and Susan could only speculate how many of them might have paused to read this lost report. As you might anticipate, every report is signed by the student clinician and supervisor, and Susan's heart sank as she observed her own name at the bottom of the second page. This grim scenario probably began as an innocent lapse in safeguarding confidential information with a partially zipped backpack, unsnapped notebook, or papers being blown unobserved from the front seat of a vehicle. But innocent or not, such lapses in safeguarding information have repercussions and consequences. The chain of events can affect the client, the supervisor, the reputation of the clinic, and the perception of the student. Susan strode into the building, her lips drawn back into a thin red line, hoping she would see the student clinician responsible for this unforgivable breakdown in protecting client confidentiality.

Information on Flash Drives Used by Students

Many students maintain information about their client(s) on flash drives in order to keep track of the information more efficiently. Students should be very cautious about using flash drives in computers outside of the university clinic or their own personal computers. Many students use flash drives that plug into the USB ports of computers. It is not uncommon for a student to have his "whole life" on that one flash drive, such as personal correspondence, classroom work, term papers, and drafts of clinical reports as well. The reason manufacturers put lanyards on those flash drives is that they are likely to be lost or misplaced because of their compact size. If you lose your flash drive you are not only losing your whole life but the lives of any clients who are mentioned in those files. In order to ensure that your client's privacy is protected while you have their reports on a flash drive, you should not use any identifying information. This may include representing their name with initials or a file number or otherwise deleting any confidential personal information. If you keep any electronic copies of your reports, make sure they are in a safe place; even better, delete those files after the information is no longer of use.

The Hard Lesson of the Hard Drive

Candace Newman was a master of using time between classes to do her homework. If she had a free hour, she would go to one of the 10 student computer labs located across the large university campus. It was a great opportunity to work on term papers for core classes in English, history, sociology, and science. It was also a chance to work on clinical reports for several clients she was seeing in practicum at the university speech and hearing clinic. Candace had diagnostic reports and midterm treatment reports that were due to be turned in to her supervisor within a week. With only 5 minutes remaining before her next class, Candace hurriedly saved her document. She had done so much work on the report that she decided to check her personal computer disk to see if the document had actually been saved. When she looked at the directory for her disk, the report was not there. So she saved the report again and confirmed that it was, in fact, on her disk. Unknown to Candace, however, her first attempt at saving the report ended up on the public computer's hard drive. Now the report, which detailed the history and personal information of Joey Dean, a child with fragile X syndrome, was available in a public computer lab for anyone to access. Maybe no one would pull the document up at all and the information would be lost in the maw of files on the hard drive. On the other hand, maybe someone would be curious about the file and access it to see what it was. Either way, Candace has planted a confidentiality time bomb that might come back to haunt her, the university clinic, her supervisor, and worst of all, Joey's family. Only time will tell.

Electronic Transmissions

Much of the communication between the university clinic and outside referral sources, allied health professionals, students and instructors, and even clients may be communicated via electronic mail (e-mail). Clinic personnel, as well as student clinicians, should be aware that this information may be read by someone other than the person or persons for whom it was intended. To this end, any and all attempts to protect our clients' privacy should be made. Identifying information such as file numbers or initials may be used instead of a client's name.

Authorization Forms

Most university clinics require clients to sign an authorization form, or "release" in order to evaluate and/or provide speech therapy services. This form is usually kept in the client's confidential file, and therefore is not subject to viewing by anyone other than clinic staff. At some university clinics that have a sliding fee schedule, prospective clients are required to report information on family size and personal income to qualify for reduced fees. Such financial information is obviously very sensitive and must be safeguarded.

Therapy Schedules

At our clinic, a comprehensive schedule of all client appointments is posted outside our front office so that anyone who needs to check the day and/or time of a therapy session can do so easily. Such a schedule should not contain client names, in that this information could be viewed by anyone entering the clinic. Instead, a file number may be used to identify each client.

Verbal Discussions

In a university setting it is not uncommon for students to communicate with one another in classes, before classes, while waiting for a client to arrive, or just walking down a corridor in the speech and hearing clinic. One of the things our students have in common is their experiences in classes and in clinical practicum. Thus, it may seem natural to discuss a client you are working with, especially if you are having a great deal of success, are frustrated due to lack of progress, or just experienced something funny during your session. While you are having these conversations you never know who will be in a position to overhear what you say. Treatment rooms are typically close to clinician areas, resulting in limited privacy and requiring you to take great care to use a volume that is appropriate and be aware of your surroundings when you are discussing clients. Although you should maintain client confidentiality by not revealing identifying information, it is okay to ask about certain procedures or goals during your academic classes. This gives you an opportunity to share with your classmates and to ensure that you understand why you are doing what you are doing.

Foot in Mouth Disease

Toni and Trisha were standing by the restroom in the clinic hallway talking about one of their clients who had not had a very productive session.

"Man, he's a brat!" Trisha complained.

"Yeah, he was terrible today. I'm sure glad I don't have to take him home," Toni replied.

Trisha laughed as she sipped her Diet Coke. "And can you believe his mother thinks there's nothing wrong with him? What's up with that?"

About that time, the mother walks out of the restroom and into the hall where the students are standing. Trisha almost chokes on her Diet Coke, as Toni, red faced, picks up her cell phone and begins a text message to her boyfriend. Mom turns and walks down the hall, obviously hurt by their rude remarks. The students look at each other in disbelief. "Man, we really messed up that time," Toni mumbles.

The next week, the mother calls the clinic and cancels her son's therapy appointment. Then, she cancels the next one, and the next one, until it's almost mid-semester. Finally, when the clinical supervisor calls to ask her if there's a problem, she says, "Yes, there certainly is, your students were saying terrible things about me and my son and I don't appreciate it one bit. I'll never come back to that clinic!"

Students should also be aware that danger of being overheard lurks outside the clinic environment as well. When you are at the mall, at a restaurant, in a nightclub, or at church you might be tempted to discuss your clinical work with a friend. If you use identifying information in these conversations there is always a chance that your client's friend, neighbor, coworker, teacher, or relative might just be at the adjacent table or strolling behind you in the mall. This is especially dangerous in small communities where people tend to know everything that is going on. *Thus, a good rule of thumb is if you have any doubt about whether to discuss information about a client, then don't!*

Audio/Video Recordings

Recording sessions is useful for accurate data collection, analysis with your supervisor, self-evaluation, or for client feedback. Students may be expected to provide their own device to record, however, most clinics offer additional resources. Small digital recorders are relatively inexpensive and easy to place close to your client. Although the sound quality is typically not as good, video recording may beneficial to glean additional detail from your sessions, especially with certain disorders. Each observation room in our clinic has a DVD player with the capability to record to the hard drive or to a CD for later review. Whether you are using a video recorder, audio recorder, or technology such as an iPad, you will need to take steps to protect your client's privacy. When listening to the recording for the purpose of data collection or analysis with your supervisor, you should choose a private environment that allows for limited access of persons not involved with your case. It is vital that after you have used the sample to gather data or use for client feedback that you delete the recording from the respective device.

In this part of the chapter, we have been discussing confidentiality as it applies to the university clinic. The next sections discuss the issue of confidentiality as it relates to medical and school settings.

MEDICAL SETTINGS

There are a number of medical settings in which speech/language evaluation and treatment take place: hospitals, long-term care facilities, skilled nursing facilities, and rehabilitation hospitals, to name a few. In our field, the term *medical setting* is generally used to refer to institutions that treat patients who have been diagnosed with any type of illness, injury, disease, or other condition that affects their speech, language, or swallowing function. These facilities are normally staffed by medical personnel such as doctors, nurses, therapists, and various other specialists. In general, a university clinic, public school, or private practice is not considered a medical setting due to the absence of any medically trained personnel.

However, there are exceptions, in that some university clinics are associated with teaching hospitals and therefore may consult with physicians or other medical professionals.

Most of the paperwork that contains client information in a medical setting is similar to paperwork seen in the university clinic (i.e., evaluation reports, therapy plans, progress notes, SOAP notes). In the university setting or private practice, each patient has a file or chart that is typically kept in the clinic office and the only professional who contributes to the chart is the SLP or audiologist. In medical facilities, the patient's chart is kept in a controlled cen-

tral location so that the many different professionals involved in the patient's care can have access to it. Therefore, it is paramount that this information is kept confidential. It is also not a good idea to discuss a patient with anyone other than those involved in his care. Often, a patient in a medical setting is noncommunicative and is therefore at the mercy of a caregiver or facility staff to protect his privacy. In this case, the student clinician should be aware of the responsibility to protect the rights of the patient. Any violation of these rights is a direct violation of HIPAA and may result in fines and or imprisonment. Being regulated by HIPAA means that you must always be conscious of the *who, what, where,* and *when*: know *who* you can talk to, *what* you can talk about, *where* you can talk about it, and *when* it is appropriate to talk about it.

John Jacobs was a distinguished attorney who had a stroke in the middle of a trial while defending his client for a murder he did not commit. Right in the middle of his introductory remarks he slumped over the table and the bailiff called 911. As a result of his stroke, Mr. Jacobs could not talk at all but could think as clearly as ever. He was incontinent and forced to wear a hospital gown that was open in the back. People he did not know wandered in and out of his room with various missions involving respiration, speech, meals, and changing IVs. He was poked and prodded by everyone from social workers to student nurses. He had a roommate who continually turned the shared television up so loud that there was no time for personal reflection. So, here was John Jacobs, attorney-at-law, who had lost every last vestige of his personal privacy. But there was one more indignity to suffer. He began to cry as he listened to a conversation between two nursing students there to change his catheter. They talked about his personal history, his son who never visited, and even the client accused of murder who was ultimately convicted.]

SCHOOL SETTINGS

The paperwork in the public schools differs significantly from the medical setting, university clinic, or private practice. This is due, in part, to the nature of the delivery of services, as well as to the federal laws that govern public schools and how they serve students with disabilities.

The Education of all Handicapped Children Act (EHA), also known as Public Law or PL 94-142, passed in 1975, mandated that all handicapped children between the ages of 3 and 21 receive a free, public education appropriate to their need, and in the least restrictive environment. In 1990, as part of its reauthorization by Congress, this law was renamed the Individuals with Disabilities Education Act or IDEA (PL 101-476). To that end, any child with a diagnosed communication disorder is covered under IDEA and entitled to free and appropriate individualized services (Haynes, Moran, & Pindzola, 2006).

Before a child can receive any special education services, including speech-language therapy, an extensive evaluation procedure is required. Once this evaluation process is complete, and it is determined that the child is eligible for special education services, an *Individualized Education Program* (IEP) must be written to meet the needs of the child. Any child with a communication disorder, who is receiving speech therapy services, will have an IEP. The IEP is unique to the school setting and is the cornerstone of a quality education for each child with a disability (U.S. Department of Education, 2005).

In most school settings, the original copy of the IEP is kept in the student's confidential file in an administrative office. Copies of the IEP are usually kept by each teacher or professional who serves the student in the special education capacity, to ensure that all of the student's goals are being addressed.

Parents may, at any time, request a copy of the IEP, at which time the school must provide such. The parent may also request that the school release a copy of the IEP to other professionals who are working with the child, such as a university speech clinic. This is the case with many of our clients, as they are receiving services from their schools as well as at our clinic. As a speech pathology practicum student in the public schools, you will be expected to implement the goals outlined for each student with whom you are assigned to work. The school SLP will usually provide a copy of the student's IEP for you to follow. For more information, go to the National Dissemination Center for Children and Youth with Disabilities (NICHCY) Web site (http://www.nichcy.org) for a detailed description of the law.

What is important to know regarding ethics and confidentiality is that any failure to implement the goals outlined in the student's IEP is a violation of federal law; therefore, each person who works with a student who has an IEP is accountable for the goals outlined therein, and this information is kept in a confidential space within the school building. Copies of a student's IEP should not be found floating around the school, or even worse, leaving the building!

Public school SLPs also keep many records in addition to the IEP. Each child will have a folder that includes various test results, treatment progress reports, weekly notes, and other forms of confidential information such as audio/video recordings. This information must be safeguarded as in any other setting until it is disposed of using appropriate methods.

We have tried to illustrate in the present chapter that there is an intimate relationship between professional ethics, protecting confidentiality, and professional communication. These relationships cross work settings and are *always* an important factor in the daily conduct of clinical work. Thus, as a student moving from one setting to another you will always carry with you a concern about patient privacy and confidentiality. It is not a question of whether confidentiality will be a major issue, because it always is. One of your first concerns in a new practicum setting is to find out how the facility handles client privacy issues and make sure you religiously adhere to those procedures.

SECTION II

Professional Written Communication

4 Diagnostic Reports

This section begins our discussion of professional written communication in speech-language pathology. What is important to know is that the diagnostic report is sometimes the first communication someone reads about a client or patient, and therefore, it must be concise yet detailed and relevant to the patient's disorder. Miller and Groher (1990) state that the best type of report "will paint a verbal picture of a clinical case and lead the reader or listener through the collection of pertinent data to a logical diagnostic conclusion" (p. 243).

If there is one concept that is important to both professional written communication and professional verbal communication it is *organization*. Without organization, one cannot write a coherent report, plan treatment goals/objectives, participate effectively in a multidisciplinary staffing, interview a parent, provide evaluation results, or counsel clients. Organization is one of the major variables that distinguishes professional from nonprofessional communication. Thus, successful beginning students as well as veteran clinicians have one thing in common: They think a lot before they write or talk.

As indicated in the title, this chapter is concerned with diagnostic report writing, and this type of report is an excellent example of why a good clinician needs to be organized. Think for a moment what happens in a diagnostic evaluation. Haynes and Pindzola (2012) illustrate that a variety of information is gathered in an evaluation. For example, you may have accumulated data in the following areas: (a) case history information, (b) prior tests and reports, (c) observation of client behavior, (d) interview findings, (e) nonstandardized testing, and (f) standardized testing. In some of these areas such as standardized testing, there may have been administration of multiple instruments. Thus, an evalua-

tion gathers multiple sources of information, and the good diagnostician must take these disparate sources of data and synthesize them to arrive at a diagnosis. In some cases the six sources of information may disagree. For instance, a child may pass a standardized language test but exhibit many errors in a spontaneous speech sample (nonstandardized testing.) The evaluator must reconcile all of these types of information to arrive at a diagnosis. Imagine if you will a desk containing case history forms, notes from a parent interview, transcripts of a communication sample, prior reports from other professionals, multiple test forms, and notes from a behavioral observation, and you will see how important organization is to approaching a diagnostic report. So far, we have only mentioned the types of data you have gathered in an assessment. The diagnostic report must not only summarize all of the types of data that have been gathered, but the clinician must arrive at a diagnosis, prognosis, suggestions for further testing, clinical management suggestions, and a rationale for referral to other professionals if appropriate. Again, as the available information is surveyed, the competent clinician is thinking about the pieces that can be used to address areas such as prognosis, treatment suggestions, and justification for referral. This requires approaching the task with an organizational structure in mind. In addition to organization, appropriate terminology is key to writing a professional diagnostic report. We illustrate some important concepts related to organization, format, and language used in diagnostic reports in the following pages. This is not meant to be a workbook for students to use in developing report writing style. We also do not take a disorder-specific approach to reporting and provide examples from the many different disorder areas in the field. There are many fine sources that do a competent job of providing practice in these areas (Middleton et al., 2001; Moon-Meyer, 2004). Our intention is to talk about the variables involved in diagnostic reporting and provide some limited examples. It is important to remember that no matter how many examples are provided in a textbook, the setting in which you are working will probably do things a bit differently than the illustrations. We think that the formats, organization process, and language are the primary determinants of professional written communication and those are what we discuss here. We also believe that it is important to illustrate diagnostic reporting as it exists across work settings at the university, medical facility, and school system.

THE ORGANIZATIONAL FRAMEWORK OF A DIAGNOSTIC REPORT

Since we have indicated that organization is so important to professional written communication, we discuss issues of format first. Not only is format important to organizing the writing of a report, it is also helpful in assembling all the information you have gathered during an evaluation. You can think of the sections of a report as boxes or bins in which you can place information you will later write about. One caveat before we begin: although there is always certain information that is "required" in a diagnostic report, various clinics may subdivide these evaluation summaries differently in terms of headings. There are many ways to slice and dice the information in a diagnostic report, and we will be presenting our own unique format in this text; keep in mind that we are providing an organizational framework to act as a general guide. Just remember that you will be using different headings depending on where you are working, but the information we mention will all be included somewhere in the report. Let's look at the typical sections in a diagnostic report:

- **Identifying Information:** This is basic demographic information such as name, age, date of birth, case/file number, gender, address, date of the evaluation, and telephone number. It is obviously important to identify the client

completely as well as when the evaluation was performed.

- **Background Information:** This includes case history information from forms, prior test results, reports from other professionals, and notes from interviewing the client, family members, or parents. The importance and type of historical information varies considerably based on the type of disorder that is present and the age of the client. For instance, neonatal, birth, and developmental history is more important for a 2-year-old than for an older child or adult. The vocational history is more important for an adult who has had a stroke than for a teenager who is still in school. Medical background is more important for clients with a medically based disorder than those with more behaviorally based problems. The clinician must look at all of the case history data and interview protocols and determine which information is the most relevant to the focus of the evaluation. This section of the diagnostic report also includes the principal reason the person was referred for the evaluation. Embedded somewhere in the background information should be a statement of why the client came for services. Although this statement is not a separate section of the report, it is important to mention the client's perspective in the background information. Utilizing the "statement of the problem" will help to focus the assessment on the topic of primary concern and will determine test selection for the evaluation.

- **Biological Bases of Communication:** What we refer to in this section is auditory acuity, structure/function of the oral mechanism, and a cursory examination of neurological integrity. Most evaluations include a hearing screening to rule out auditory acuity problems or to justify referral to an audiologist for a full evaluation.

  A statement of the results of the audiological screening goes in this section and usually provides information on the frequencies screened and the attenuation level of the audiometer. Especially in cases where motoric or structural abnormalities are suspected, we perform an oral-peripheral examination, which tests the structure and function of the oral mechanism. We also note any possible neurological symptoms such as paralysis, weakness, drooling, deficits in fine and gross motor skill, or client reports of seizures or head injury.

This section can be quite brief if there are no remarkable findings. Obviously, the more abnormalities that are noted in structure or function of the speech mechanism, the longer this section will become.

■ **Basic Communication Processes of Language, Articulation, Voice/Resonance, and Fluency That Are Within Normal Limits:** When a person undergoes an evaluation for a possible communication disorder, it is assumed that the diagnostician has examined *all basic processes of communication*. For instance, we do not know that a client referred for an articulation problem does not have a language disorder as well. Thus, it is imperative that at some point in the evaluation the clinician take the time to assess, if only informally, the four areas of language, articulation, voice/resonance, and fluency. In most cases we will not administer formal tests in the four basic areas because we can see from nonstandardized tasks such as conversation that there are no significant problems. For example, a child referred for misarticulations can be judged to exhibit normal vocal characteristics and fluency from listening to a conversational sample. Especially in the university practicum setting, students might be asked to administer tests for several of the basic communication processes for the purpose of gaining experience in test administration. However, in other settings, formal testing of all areas of communication is often omitted and not reported on because they are not areas of major concern. In those cases, a clinician might not test articulation in a case that was referred for fluency, especially if no misarticulations were noted in spontaneous conversation. The bottom line here is that the diagnostic report must address, however briefly, the basic areas of communication to show that we have considered each of these as an area of possible communication disorder. This could be a brief

statement such as, "With regard to age and gender, no abnormalities were noted in the client's vocal quality, resonance, articulation, or fluency."

■ **Diagnostic Test Results Focusing on the Area(s) of Concern:** The bulk of the diagnostic report will involve detailing the test results on the patient's area of major concern. If that concern is a child language disorder, we will be reporting the results of many standardized tests and the results of different analyses of a language sample (e.g., mean length of utterance, type-token ratio, syntactic complexity, grammatical errors, pragmatic difficulties). If the concern is a fluency disorder, we will be administering and reporting many measurements of overt behaviors (e.g., frequency and type of dysfluency) and indicators of covert dimensions related to stuttering (such as feelings, attitudes, avoidances). A person whose primary concern is hoarseness will be administered many behavioral and instrumental measures of phonation during a variety of tasks ranging from prolonging vowels to connected speech. It only makes sense that the diagnostic report will devote the most space and focus to the topic of major concern.

■ **Clinical Impressions and Prognosis:** In this section of a report, the clinician interprets the different test results and background information to arrive at a diagnosis and prognosis. If a disorder is present, the nature and severity of the disorder should be described as well as any pertinent medical history. The prognosis for improving function should also be documented, using age, medical and communication diagnoses, family support, level of motivation, and cognitive functioning as a guide. Prognosis can be defined in terms of good, fair, poor, or guarded. This section is longer when there is disagreement among the different types of clinical data because the clinician has to explain discrepancies in results.

■ **Summary and Recommendations:** This section is the most frequently read portion of a diagnostic report, especially by busy professionals. The evaluation is briefly summarized and specific recommendations for treatment, no treatment, or referral are detailed.

The organization of a diagnostic report, whether written for an adult or child client, will usually contain information from the sections presented above.

While an evaluation done in any work setting is concerned with the same basic information we have just described, diagnostic reporting across work settings is not exactly the same. The principal difference revolves around the length of the reports. Reports in medical and school settings tend to be shorter due to (a) limitations in the use of narrative explanations and (b) report forms that limit length due to use of check boxes to indicate the presence/absence of abnormality, or a limited space allocated to note test scores. We discuss these versions of diagnostic reports in later sections.

UNIVERSITY CLINIC

Length, Content, and Format

As you probably know by now, the university clinic requires students to write detailed reports summarizing the evaluation process. In the university setting, most students begin by learning to write long narrative reports that in some cases may be five or more pages in length, depending on the type of case. It should be noted that while the report is several pages, the point is not to make the report as lengthy as possible but to be inclusive of all pertinent information that reflects the client's communication skills and your recommendations. One reason these reports are longer than in other settings is that students are often asked to administer tests that are not particularly necessary for diagnosis but are selected to give the student experience with testing. A second reason these reports are long is that students need to gain experience with professional writing. At some point in your career you might be asked to write a detailed report as part of a legal proceeding or to explain a very complicated case to another professional to whom a client is referred. In these instances, knowing how to provide clinical detail in a professional manner is important. Another reason

for longer reports is that most university clinics perform comprehensive speech and language evaluations, sometimes lasting up to 2 hours. Some other settings may have evaluation time slots that extend only 20 to 30 minutes. You can simply get more testing done in 2 hours, and then you have to report the results. A final reason for the longer reports is that in the training setting, we can ask students to do more time-intensive tasks such as transcribing language samples and analyzing video recordings of play behaviors. These are important skills for students to develop. Even though such analyses represent the highest level of validity and expertise in our field, they may not be done in medical or school settings. In general, a person in a private practice, school system, or medical facility may not have the time to perform such an in-depth evaluation. However, because the university clinic is a training facility, students may be exposed to the full gamut of evaluation procedures. Thus, in the university training program you will be writing the longest of your clinical reports and you will need to learn how to pare them down in other settings. It is better, however, to know the long version before you move into more abbreviated clinical writing. As Shipley and McAfee (2008) point out, the consolation for you, the student, is that once you graduate and practice professionally, you will be able to pick and choose aspects you like from all the different models and develop your own unique style of writing.

Now we address the content of the report in a university setting. We gather so much information in a diagnostic evaluation that it is sometimes difficult to determine what is important and what is not. So, what are the ingredients of a good report? How do you get to a logical diagnostic conclusion? Let's start with first things first. A thorough description of the patient's case history is imperative. I want to learn as much as I can about this person in the first paragraph of this report. Just as if I were reading a good book, I want something to draw me in, keep me interested, and be informative. Rambling, unimportant information is not going to keep my attention, but concise, detailed, relevant information will. Identifying information such as name, address, telephone number, and date of birth are required and it is critical to insure this information is correct. Sections such as background information and statement of the problem are not always straightforward and the clinician will have to make some judgment calls on certain issues. For instance, is it more important that Jimmy likes to play soccer, or that he "can't remember anything" since he fell and hit his head on the driveway? We would vote for the head injury. It is always good to preserve the patient's or parent's statement of the problem. This is the statement that helps to guide the evaluation toward the topic of immediate concern. So, if you ask a parent why she brought her son in for an evaluation, she might say, "John has been struggling with saying his words. It's like he gets stuck and you can see the frustration on his face. I'm worried that he is beginning to stutter." That is the kind of quote that belongs in a diagnostic report because it helps to focus the evaluation and justify all of the tests and tasks you performed to assess fluency under various conditions. Speech pathology practicum students often make the mistake of not including enough pertinent information or, on the other hand, adding information that is unnecessary. A good rule of thumb is to report any information that you feel could impact speech, language, or swallowing function and describe it so that it makes sense.

Regarding other data to be mentioned in a diagnostic report, clearly the format sections we mentioned earlier will dictate the inclusion of certain types of information. Obviously, test results from standardized and nonstandardized information are important to include. After providing scores from standardized tests, it is vital to provide an explanation for what the scores reveal. After reporting test results, the diagnostic report should relate clinical impressions and prognosis, summarize the findings, and make recommendations or referrals. Usually the reporting of scores or behavioral data involves listing numerical information and perhaps some behavioral description. Clinical impressions and recommendations tend to be more narrative in nature but still based firmly on the historical information, test results, and behavioral observation.

Writing Style

In this section we get down to the nuts and bolts of professional written communication and discuss terminology and common errors students commit in clinical reports.

> *Student 1:* "I hate writing reports because my supervisor always changes everything I write."
>
> *Student 2:* "Yeah, I know what you mean. Mine looks like it's bleeding to death when I get it back from my supervisor—red everywhere!"
>
> *Student 1:* "She never likes the way I say things. It's like she thinks I'm stupid or something."

Has this scenario happened to you? More than likely, if you are a student in a university SLP program, it has. What is it about reports that makes them so difficult? Why is it that certain things have to be said a "certain way" or they are wrong? The truth of the matter is, what is written by students is not always wrong; it is just that reports are different when written by different people and across work settings. The format, style, length, and degree of detail needed for a diagnostic report varies across settings, university programs, and sometimes even supervisors in the same setting (Shipley & McAfee, 2008).

Some 30 years ago an article entitled, "The Agony of Report Writing: A New Look at an Old Problem" (Haynes & Hartman, 1975) addressed this. Interestingly, this article is still quoted extensively in the most recent textbooks dealing with professional writing (Middleton et al., 2001; Moon-Meyer, 2004). The reason that the article remains relevant is not that it was particularly groundbreaking or prescient, but because clinical writing still inflicts a good deal of pain on students in training, just as it always has. In that article two areas were outlined that still have the imprint of clinical relevance to students. One area was a professional terminology generator that provided examples of the kinds of terms used in clinical reports. There is a certain type of language used in professional communication and there is no reason to keep it a secret from our students. In the present text (Appendix A), the terminology generator has been modified to include general terms from specific disorder areas and updated terms. Students can use the professional terminology generator in several ways. First, when you are searching for a term to use in writing a report and you cannot think of one, you can look at the items in Appendix A for possible examples to use. Second, you can use the generator to reduce redundancy in reports. For example, there is redundancy in the following: "The client was not stimulable for any error phonemes.

The client responded well to phonetic placement of bilabial stop consonants." Choosing another term to refer to the client would reduce redundancy in the two sentences ("The client was not stimulable for any error phonemes; however, he responded well to phonetic placement of bilabial stop consonants."). There are many ways to say that a patient "has" a particular condition (e.g., *shows, exhibits, manifests, demonstrates, displays,* etc.) and you do not have to redundantly use the same term in every sentence.

There are also "professional tone words" in the generator that are often the variable that separates professional clinical communication from everyday speech. We encourage you to incorporate professional terminology in your reports from the beginning and not rely on your clinical supervisor to change what you have written to increase its professional tone.

Common Errors

Many sources discuss common mistakes that students make in their early report writing (Haynes & Hartman, 1975; Haynes & Pindzola, 2012; Knepflar, 1978; Meitus, 1991; Moore, 1969; Shipley & McAfee, 2008). We feel that these frequent errors should not be kept a secret from students, but should be mentioned so that they can be proactive in clinical writing. Some of the following are errors mentioned in the above references:

1. **Redundancy:** This refers to the use of the same terms within a sentence and across abutting sentences. Redundancy can also refer to repetition of the same concept or idea. For example, the following sentences basically say the same thing: *The results of this evaluation suggest that Joey will have little difficulty in correcting his articulation problem. Joey's prognosis for improving his articulation skills is good.*

2. **Wordiness:** Every attempt should be made to state diagnostic information in the most economical way possible. Reports are no place for wordy descriptions. This is why we use professional terminology. Instead of saying, "The client could not produce the phonemes that were in error even with multiple trials of maximum

multisensory stimulation and modeling," it is enough to say, "The client was not stimulable for any errored phonemes despite maximum cueing."

3. **Lack of Professional Terminology:** As we illustrate in the terminology generator in Appendix A there are certain professional terms that are typically used in reports. Common errors include using "I" instead of "the clinician" and using "sounds" for "phonemes."

4. **Lack of Objectivity and Not Separating Fact from Opinion:** Reports should include objective information and not unsubstantiated assumptions on the part of the clinician. Reasonable interpretation of test scores is fairly objective in terms of characterizing a client's performance in relation to standard scores. A person who scores 2 standard deviations below the mean could easily be considered to exhibit a disorder in the area tested. If we are talking about parent reports, we should couch these with phrases such as "the parent reported . . . the mother stated." If we are talking about our own opinions, this should be stated as such ("It is the opinion of the examiner that Mary is not highly motivated for treatment."). This should be followed by a description of behaviors that support the clinician's observation such as the client's reluctance to enter the treatment room, crying when entering the clinical setting, and screaming, "I hate coming here," at the beginning of every session.

5. **Lack of Organization and Sequence:** Make sure that the appropriate information is included in the correct section of your report. For example, do not bring up history information in the clinical impressions section. A report should be organized in such a way that it flows from background information to test results to clinical impressions and finally to recommendations.

6. **Ambiguity:** A sentence such as, "The client did not perform well on the motor speech tasks," does not really tell us anything specific about performance. The client may not have tried very hard on the task or might have shown serious motoric deficits. A sentence such as, "The client has articulation problems," does not tell us anything specific about the client's performance. Providing the most specific details regarding the

client's performance is important in relaying the most accurate picture of the client for anyone who might read the report. A sentence such as, "The client exhibited consistent final consonant deletion which decreased his intelligibility to 60% for unfamiliar content." provides the reader with a more thorough account of the client's speech and language.

7. **Tense Errors:** Typically, the case history portion of the report is written in past tense. Later, when discussing clinical impressions and recommendations, you can switch to more active sentence constructions, since you are talking about the present and the future.

8. **Spelling and Typographical Errors:** In this age of spell-checkers and grammatical screeners in word processing programs, there is no excuse for spelling and typographical errors for clinical reports. Just remember that your spell checker may not recognize clinical jargon that you have included in your report so you may need to consult another resource such as your textbook for the correct spelling.

9. **Wrong Use of Abbreviations:** While it is acceptable to use an abbreviation in a report, it should always be initially defined the first time it is used. A child might be administered the Goldman-Fristoe Test of Articulation (GFTA-2). If it is defined, as in the previous sentence, then it is all right to use GFTA-2 in later portions of the report.

10. **Use of Contractions and Informal Language:** Reports are no place to use contracted forms (e.g., *can't, won't, we'll, he'll,* etc.). Most authorities recommend using the fully formed versions of words that are amenable to contraction. Also, the use of informal, shortened versions of words such as "rehab" for rehabilitation is typically not recommended. Obviously, slang terminology such as "freaked out" or "messed up" is not acceptable in reports.

Do Not Forget Your Audience

Clinical reports end up in the hands of many different types of people. It is not possible to write a report that will be equally understood by your colleagues in SLP and a parent with limited educational experience. Another professional (e.g., psychologist, classroom teacher) may not understand terms that are unique to communication disorders, but if they are truly professional they will have encountered our terms before or will look them up. Certainly, when we receive reports from psychologists, they do not hesitate to use terminology unique to psychology. One solution would be to write the report to the lowest common denominator of audiences and remove all professional terms. This would help laypeople understand the report, but it would marginalize our profession. We have worked for many years to raise our profession to the same standard as other health-related professions, and part of that involves our style of reporting. One does not see psychologists, educational evaluation specialists, physical therapists, physicians, and occupational therapists write reports without professional language. If that were the case, a psychologist would have to explain IQ and testing methods in the report so that it would be understandable to laypersons. There are, however, schools of thought in report writing that suggest we should generate reports that are "parent-friendly" or "family-friendly," omitting professional terms or including definitions and explanations of concepts referred to in the report. In some ways this is good for the family, but it makes our profession seem less than it is. A family-friendly report certainly would not represent our profession as well if sent to a psychologist or physician. Discipline-specific terms exist because they allow us to refer to phenomena in an efficient and professional way. Thus, it is important for you to remember where the report is going to be sent and who is primarily going to profit from reading it. If it is going in the university clinic file, it should be written professionally for another SLP. If it is going to a public school SLP, again, it should be written professionally. If the report is going to a professional from another discipline you should consider this while writing and define terms you feel may be unique. In medical or school settings, however, most people who work there share common terminology and freely use medical or educational terms because they communicate most efficiently. One compromise is that some clinics write reports for the clinical file and then write a separate letter to parents summarizing the results of the evaluation in less technical terms. There is no one way to write reports that has been agreed upon by clinics and work settings throughout the country. So, our best advice is to consider your primary audience and be as professional as possible. In some cases it may mean drafting several versions of your findings for various audiences either in the form of alternate reports or summary letters for parents. Ultimately, there must be a balance between communicating information and communicating professionally. One thing is certain: You should not buy *The Big Book of Vocabulary* and learn words such as *magnanimous* or *obfuscation* and then amaze your colleagues by placing them in a clinical report. According to Haynes and Pindzola (2008), "A diagnostic report is no place to display your learning or to parade a large vocabulary. Pedantic reports are misunderstood or unread" (p. 377).

In Appendices B and C we provide examples of each section of a diagnostic report, based on the evaluation of a child and an adult. Through your graduate training, you will be exposed to various types of assessment based on specific disorders; therefore, we will not provide examples of a diagnostic report for every disorder in this text. In the next sections we will expand our discussion of diagnostic reporting to other settings beyond the university.

MEDICAL SETTINGS

A diagnostic report in a hospital, nursing home, or rehabilitation facility will most likely look very different from a report in the university clinic. The most noticeable differences will be the amount of information included and the format. In many medical facilities, your documentation will involve checking boxes, filling in short blanks, or writing a short description on a computer generated form that other disciplines may be writing on as well. In some settings, you may simply record a number to represent the patient's abilities. We have included several examples of diagnostic reporting forms from a medical setting in Appendices D through F.

Most students who complete a practicum in a medical setting are initially thrilled when they see how "easy" these diagnostic forms are to fill out.

The only drawback is you have to know exactly what information is relevant before you can accurately complete the form—this is where your practice in writing lengthy diagnostic reports comes in handy. You have already practiced figuring out what information is most pertinent and reporting it in a narrative format; now, you can apply that information to the new format. It's easy, right? Not so fast. Many of the supervisors in the medical setting that we talked to while researching the present textbook told us that students still have difficulty "filling out the form." What we learned is that students are still tentative about which boxes to check or that they are not very familiar with the medical terminology. To help you in this area, we provide a list of the most commonly used medical terms and symbols in Appendix K.

While knowledge of terminology will be of some assistance to beginning students, familiarity with terms alone will not alleviate your tentativeness as your pen or mouse hovers over a series of check boxes. Your greatest ally will be a logical organization of your case history data and assessment data and clear thinking about the results of the evaluation. The same procedures you went through in the university clinic are important to use in understanding the case, no matter how brief the report format. If you must choose between *aphasia* and *motor speech disorder*, you still must have thought through the evidence from your evaluation before checking the appropriate box. The important thing is that you understand *why* you are checking a particular box on a diagnostic form.

In most cases, a diagnostic report in a hospital, nursing home, or rehabilitation facility will include the same basic information (give or take a few sections) as a diagnostic report you would write in a university clinic. Reports may be written by hand in the chart or, if you are at a more technologically advanced facility, you will sit down at a computer, open a software program, and point and click your way to describing your patient's speech, language or swallowing problem. You then click "print" and your diagnostic report is ready!

Do not get too far ahead of yourself, though. It is still very important that you have adequate knowledge of what is important in order to be a good diagnostic reporter. As long as you use the information provided thus far, you should be on the right track.

SCHOOL SETTINGS

Reports in the public schools vary greatly from the typical report that you would see in a medical setting, private practice, or university clinic. The information gleaned from a diagnostic evaluation may not be written down in a standard diagnostic format, as has been discussed in the previous sections, although we have seen this done in certain states. We have found that in many school systems, once the evaluation is completed, the information is compiled, discussed by the IEP team, and then transferred to an eligibility form. What you as a practicum student in the schools will see is this eligibility form. The form will include all areas of assessment, dates and names of the assessments, as well as the results. In addition, the student's strengths and needs will be included.

An example of an eligibility form is included in Appendix G. According to school personnel, determining strengths and needs is one of the most difficult tasks for speech pathology practicum students. Thus, the challenge of diagnostic reports in the schools is not so much in reporting the test findings, but in determining the needs of each child, based on a comprehensive evaluation.

Let's talk about what this comprehensive evaluation entails. In most public school systems, you are required to administer at least two formal assessments in language and one formal assessment in speech. The language scores will then be calculated, and, based on the standard score, it will be determined if a child is eligible for services. Eligibility determination differs by state and in some cases even by school system within the same state. Typically, a language or articulation standard score must be more than 1.5 to 2 standard deviations (SD) below the mean in order for a child to qualify for services in either speech or language disorders. Most school systems require the SLP to administer a comprehensive language assessment, one that tests both receptive and expressive language. Then, if a child shows a deficit in expressive language, for instance, the

SLP must administer a formal assessment that specifically targets expressive language. According to IDEA, informal assessments can also be made part of the evaluation process. This is especially important in cases where a student may pass standardized tests but evidence errors in a spontaneous speech sample. Although informal assessments may not be considered by some school systems when determining if a child has a language delay, obtaining a language sample can be an invaluable resource in helping to "nail down" even more specific areas of deficit in children who are language impaired. Parents also have the right to seek a second opinion from a source outside the school system if they disagree with the determination of eligibility or diagnosis of their child (Haynes, Moran, & Pindzola, 2006). Also, it is important to remember that there is a significant difference between arriving at a diagnosis and determining eligibility. Diagnosis involves using standardized and nonstandardized testing to determine the existence of a communication disorder and make specific recommendations for treatment. Eligibility determination is largely an administrative operation that allows school systems to select with whom they will work. These two operations are quite different. One can have a communication disorder and may not qualify for services in the school system if it determines the disorder has no impact on educational progress or if test scores do not indicate enough of a deficit to meet criteria for eligibility.

Formal assessment is also important when evaluating a child with a fluency disorder in order to determine if the severity of the disorder warrants intervention; however, this assessment should not be limited to fluency counts, percentage of stuttered syllables, or other formal measures of severity alone. Assessment of stuttering should include discussion of the child's attitudes and emotions about her stuttering and consider the overall impact of the disorder on participation in her life (Yarrus, 2007).

At times, a child will be identified as having a voice problem during the course of a speech, language, or fluency evaluation. Because this is a subjective judgment by the speech-language clinician, it may be necessary to refer the child for medical follow-up with an ear, nose, and throat specialist (ENT). Often, the school clinician will initiate a vocal abuse awareness and/or vocal hygiene program that will be included in the child's speech goals.

Once the evaluations are finished, an eligibility form is completed. Each assessment that has been administered to the child (and the completion date) is listed, along with a description of the child's strengths and needs in each area. From there, goals are developed that target deficit areas (whether in speech, language, voice, or fluency) and benchmarks are established that will enable the SLP to help the child meet goals in the most timely and efficient manner. Figure 4–1 gives a better idea of how the diagnostic process works in the public schools.

This chapter would not be complete without a mention of computerized report writing. As you can well imagine, there are software programs for generating almost any type of document that exists. This is also true for the field of speech-language pathology. Many hospitals, private practices, and school agencies now use computer programs to generate diagnostic reports, treatment reports (see Chapter 5), progress notes, and IEPs. There are many programs available in today's market, and sometimes knowing which one to choose can be challenging. Middleton et al. (2001, p. 69) remind us, "It is important when considering report writing software to evaluate the quality of reports as well as their applicability for each individual clinical circumstance." In the public schools, it has become commonplace for special educators, administrators, teachers, and SLPs to use IEP software. There are a myriad of programs available for generating IEPs, and depending on the state you are in, you may or may not be exposed to these. It is good to know about these programs and the ways that computer generated reports may increase the efficiency of documentation of service delivery.

It is important to remember, however, that *you* are still the clinician and the computer programs referred to above cannot think for you. This is especially critical in report writing programs that actually generate sentences based on information the clinician is prompted to provide. Always proofread the computer-generated report for accuracy and do not let the algorithms put words in your mouth, especially if they could be misinterpreted by those reading the report. No matter how a report is generated, it is always the responsibility of the clinician to insure clarity and accuracy.

Figure 4–1. Diagnostic process in the school setting.

In closing, what is most important for you, the practicum student, to realize is that thorough assessment of the patient or client, along with a clear description of the results and implications of that assessment, is the first step in providing the most efficacious plan of care. In order to function as a competent provider of services, you must begin with an accurate, professional, and meaningful description of your patient/client's needs.

5 Documenting Treatment Planning: Goals, Objectives, Data, and Rationales

Speech-language pathology is an extremely diverse and ever-changing profession that encompasses a vast array of disorders and individuals from infants to geriatrics. Clinicians are beginning to specialize in the assessment and treatment of various disorders; so much so that certification in specific areas is becoming commonplace. At the same time, ongoing research, in the form of evidence-based practice (EBP), is opening doors to new avenues of treatment and new ways of understanding disorders of communication. Thus, the field of communication disorders is constantly changing. It may be daunting to you, a student, to imagine becoming competent in every area of this diverse field. However, it should be of some comfort to know that where there is change, there is also some consistency. What does *not* change is the fact that treatment of communication disorders must be planned, based on a thorough assessment, executed in a way that is efficacious and practical, and reported in a meaningful way. This chapter focuses on the process of establishing measurable goals and objectives and providing the rationales to back them up. We focus on each of the various work settings and the way in which treatment planning is similar and different for each. We also define a rationale and discuss why it is important to be able to explain why we make clinical decisions. Accurate data collection is paramount and it's importance is detailed as well. The reason we address these issues in a textbook on professional communication is that you will be asked repeatedly to communicate goals and rationales verbally and in many types of reports, including treatment plans, progress summaries, and other forms as part of your clinical training.

In your coursework you have no doubt dealt with the concept that thought and mental organization underlie the language we use to communicate ideas. Thus, your verbal and written communication is organized by how you think about the topic of interest. We raised this issue in the previous chapter on diagnostic reports by saying that *organization* is key to developing professional clinical writing. In the case of treatment efforts, you must develop a principled way of thinking about goals and procedures before you can coherently talk or write about them. The process of thinking about a client's long-term goal provides you with an ultimate target that will be achieved when you dismiss the person from treatment. The short-term goals are the steps that you follow in a systematic way to approach the target. In psychology, this is known as successive (or progressive) approximation. We cannot expect that a client will achieve the long-term goal right away, but rather will move toward it in a systematic fashion. In fact, the whole concept of successive approximation is based on the notion that one cannot achieve long-term objectives without accomplishing short-term goals. They are the baby steps that allow a person to build competence on one level so that he can perform at higher levels. Clinicians must put a great deal of thought into identifying and sequencing goals of treatment so that they represent a hierarchy of difficulty leading to the ultimate long-term objective. If you have thought through the process, you will have much less difficulty writing a treatment plan or explaining what you are doing with a client to parents, family members, or observers of your treatment sessions.

In the first part of this chapter, we discuss goals and objectives and why they are an integral part of speech and language therapy reporting. We should note that our purpose in this chapter is not to provide examples of goal writing for every disorder that you might encounter in clinical practicum. Our mission here is to talk about the process of goal writing and how it drives your professional communication about the client. Figure 5–1 shows the components involved in writing goals for a particular client. One component is your background knowledge gained from academic coursework. For example, you need information about normal development of the communication parameter that is affected in the client you are working with to determine the order in which normally developing individuals acquire the skill. This can be a powerful indicator of the difficulty involved in skill acquisition, and normal development is often used as a guideline in ordering treatment goals. Another aspect of background knowledge is information about the particular disorder your client exhibits. For example, if it is phonology, you should know about the types of phonological errors commonly seen in children with disorders. You should also know about assessment and treatment procedures for use in treating phonological impairments. Thus, there is no substitute for background knowledge in writing goals because this information helps you to select target behaviors, sequence them in order of difficulty, and choose appropriate tasks to use in the conduct of therapy.

A second component in writing goals is specific knowledge of your client's current level of perfor-

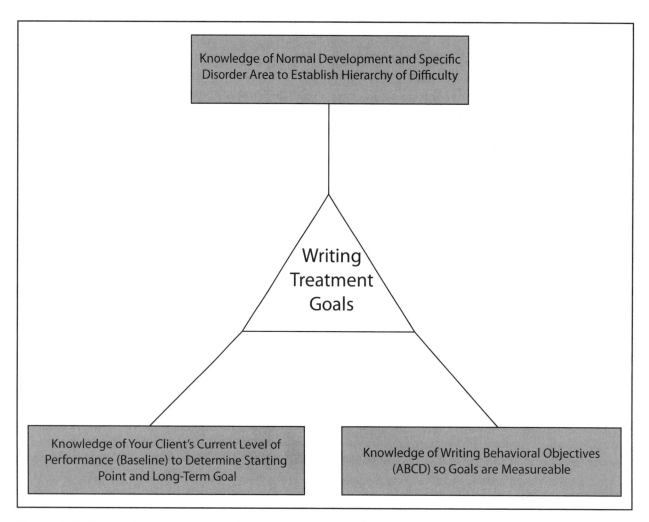

Figure 5–1. Prerequisite components of writing treatment goals.

mance and cognitive abilities. This again emphasizes the importance of a thorough evaluation so that you will know exactly what the client can and cannot do with regard to phonological production, as in the previous example. The results of an evaluation may also impact your setting of long-term goals. For example, if a multidisciplinary evaluation revealed that your client has cognitive limitations such as mental retardation, a long-term goal of 100% intelligibility in complex sentences may not be realistic. The third component of writing goals is the basic process in which we specify certain information as part of crafting observable, measurable behavioral objectives. You should be able to see from Figure 5–1 that if any component is missing, the clinician will be at a loss to develop appropriate goals. It should also be apparent that a single chapter on writing goals cannot address all three components in Figure 5–1. We focus only on the mechanics of writing behavioral objectives in this chapter and leave it to you to combine classroom information with these guidelines to arrive at measurable goals. For additional guidelines for the components of a behavioral objective, see Appendix P. We also illustrate how these goals are similar and different in their appearance across practicum settings.

WHAT ARE LONG-TERM AND SHORT-TERM GOALS?

After an evaluation is completed, and before beginning a program of intervention, you will have to establish the goals that you will be working toward in therapy. The essence of intervention planning is the determination of long-term intervention goals and the development of procedures by which to achieve them. Klein and Moses (1994) define an intervention goal as "a potential achievement by an individual with a speech-language dysfunction directed toward the improvement of speech-language performance" (p. 3). The first step in planning treatment involves setting long-term goals, which will stipulate what you ultimately want your client to achieve. Once your long-term goals are established, you can then go on to the second step, which is to prioritize target behaviors that will lead the client toward achievement of the long-term goals.

An example of a long-term goal is:

■ The client will produce all age-appropriate phonemes in spontaneous connected speech outside the therapeutic environment with 90% accuracy.

An example of a short-term goal is:

■ The client will spontaneously produce /t/ in the initial position of words while looking at picture cards with 90% accuracy in the clinical setting.

According to Klein and Moses (1994) a short-term goal is "a linguistic achievement that has been given priority within a hierarchy of achievements required for the realization of the long-term goal" (p. 130). In other words, the short-term goals are made up of *specific* behaviors you want to target in therapy that will enable your client to achieve long-term goals. In the previous example, the short-term goal of "correct production of /t/ in words" is the first step in helping the client to produce age-appropriate phonemes that will improve overall intelligibility. The term *given priority* means that you have chosen these behaviors to be worked on first, assuming they will result in the most effective and efficient course of treatment. Which target behaviors are given priority should be influenced by ease of teaching; natural sequence of current behaviors/prerequisite behaviors, and what will result in an increase in the client's function. It is worth your time to communicate with the client and/or their family to determine which goals will be most motivating for them and those that might be functional for the client, meaning relevant for their daily life. You can imagine that a client and their family might have increased interest in targeting a behavior in which they will see carryover into daily routines.

As the name implies, short-term refers to a definitive period of time. Obviously, we would not want to generate all of the possible steps leading from the client's current level of performance to the achievement of a long-term goal. That might entail scores of individual steps if you consider all of the different levels of language ranging from phoneme production to complex sentences, and all of the levels from imitative tasks to spontaneous conversation. Not only would this be unwieldy, but it would not take into account the possibility of generalization and spontaneous learning on the part of the client, which might make it possible to skip planned levels of training. Thus, we limit our short-term goals to a well-defined window of time. For example, the amount of time designated for achieving a short-term goal and the number of short-term goals are often determined by where the therapy is taking place. In the university clinic, the goal may be for a semester; in a hospital, it may be for a few days or a week; and in a long-term care facility, it may last until the patient's insurance stops paying for services. Generally, in these situations, the insurance company will stipulate how long the patient is able to receive therapy. For instance, they might say 30 visits or not to exceed 8 weeks. It is, however, important to know that the procedure for choosing your short-term goals is virtually the same across work settings and various lengths of treatment. The bottom line is that you need to think about how many short-term steps the client can realistically accomplish in the time frame allotted (semester, school year, a month in a rehabilitation hospital, or a week in acute care). Pertinent factors in determining how many short-term objectives to target for each given period of time include current level of functioning, severity and type of the disorder, behavior, the frequency and duration of therapy, and participation and compliance with a home program.

Another important issue to consider is that most often a client will have more than a single short-term goal. Short-term goals often interlock with one another and they represent different facets of the same underlying aspect of client growth. For example, a child who has a limited expressive lexicon of 40 words at age 3 might have a short-term objective (STO) of increasing lexicon size to 75 words. This client might also have a STO of increasing mean length of utterance (MLU) from 1.0 to 2.0. To increase this MLU, specific types of word combinations might be targeted such as basic operations of reference (more

+ X, that + X, allgone + X) and two-term semantic relations (agent + action; action + object). Thus, this child has several STOs that involve increasing expressive lexicon size, increasing MLU, increasing use of basic operations of reference, and increasing use of certain two-term semantic relations. When you think about it, all four STOs relate to teaching the child to use multiword utterances. All of this could potentially be accomplished in a university setting during the course of one semester.

WHAT IS A BEHAVIORAL OBJECTIVE?

A behavioral objective is a statement that describes the intended target behavior in an observable and measurable way. The behavioral objective is the staple of everyday treatment planning. Think of the behavioral objective as an instruction manual or a blueprint for how to conduct a therapy session. Just as with building a house, it is difficult to get started without the blueprint. Similarly, without the instruction manual, you would not know how to put together a bookcase, for example, or a child's swing set. You must have a plan for how to conduct a therapy session, and your objectives are your plan. Those objectives not only dictate your behavior in the treatment session but also how you talk and write about what you do in professional communication.

The first thing to remember about objectives is they must be something you can both observe and measure. In order to accomplish this, the clinician must identify what the client is expected to do, under what conditions, and with what degree of success. Owens, Metz, and Farinella (2011, p. 96) suggest that the letters ABCD are helpful in remembering the format for writing behavioral objectives:

A. **Audience:** Who is expected to demonstrate the behavior?
B. **Behavior:** What is the observable and measurable behavior?
C. **Condition:** What is the context or condition of the behavior?
D. **Degree:** What is the targeted degree of success?

With this "blueprint" you should be able to write a measurable objective for any behavior that you wish to target in therapy.

Example 1:

A. Billy
B. will spontaneously produce /s/
C. in the initial position of words while naming pictures
D. with 90% accuracy over 3 consecutive sessions.

Example 2:

A. Karen
B. will include narrative elements of setting and character
C. in a spontaneous story in response to sequence pictures
D. in 3 out of 5 opportunities during a therapy session.

Example 3:

A. Robyn
B. will increase the number of spontaneous words to request or label
C. during 15 minutes of structured play with the clinician
D. to a minimum of 20 single words.

Example 4:

A. James
B. will utilize smooth, controlled speech
C. with an unfamiliar listener inside the therapy room during a 5-minute conversation
D. in 50% of communicative opportunities.

As long as you have identified your client's deficits, based on a thorough assessment, you should be able to apply this formula to create appropriate objectives for treatment. Note that in the above examples we have specified the stimulus (pictures), the task (spontaneous) and the response (/s/ phoneme in words; story production). Degree may be measured in time, number, or frequency. These are critical components to include in objectives. In some settings, you may add a time period to short-term

objectives, such as, "By the end of the semester" or, on an IEP you may stipulate a month and year such as, "By May 2013."

Selected words to *avoid* in writing behavioral objectives:

Understand, listen, enjoy, think, know, review, develop an appreciation, like, comprehend, feel, learn, become able, attain, grasp, memorize, acquire, discover, discern, assimilate, digest, grasp, perceive, recognize

We suggest avoiding such words because they are *not measurable and observable.*

Selected words that may be useful in writing behavioral objectives:

Define, describe, identify, label, list, match, name, outline, select, state, explain, give example, paraphrase, summarize, compute, predict, produce, show, solve, use, diagram, differentiate, discriminate, distinguish, recall, illustrate, outline, select, categorize, compose, organize, plan, rewrite, write, tell, compare, contrast, justify, interpret, ask, choose, follow directions, give, locate, point to, sit, reply, take turns, answer, comply, greet, perform, read, initiate, share, work, combine

---

WHAT IS A RATIONALE?

One of the most important questions you can ever ask yourself, in any situation, is, "Why do I do what I do?" This is certainly true in the field of SLP with intervention planning. Establishing a rationale for your treatment protocol is extremely important, possibly one of the most important aspects of your training. So, that being said, let's talk about rationales and how they are used in therapy.

Webster's Dictionary defines *rationale* as "an underlying principle." If you look up the word *rationale* in a thesaurus, you will see words such as *justification, basis, validation, reasoning,* and *logic.* As this applies to speech-language treatment, you must have a basis, or reasoning, for what you do with your clients. The rationale for your treatment may be based upon several factors, most of which come about through ongoing research—there is scientific evidence that proves various treatment techniques are effective. Evidence-based practice (EBP) is a "hot button" issue in our field at this time, and you will most likely hear this term referred to frequently throughout your professional career (Haynes & Johnson, 2009). In 2004, ASHA's executive board stated that the goal of EBP is the integration of: (a) clinical expertise, (b) best current evidence, and (c) client values to provide high-quality services reflecting the interests, values, needs, and choices of the individuals we serve (ASHA, 2004). Kamhi et al. (2009) state that EBP is continuous and is "a dynamic integration of ever-evolving clinical expertise and external evidence in day-to-day practice." When you use EBP to determine your course of action with a client, you will be communicating not only your goal of structuring therapy goals with the latest research and your previous experiences, but also with the client's individual needs at the forefront. In essence, all of the therapy techniques that are being used today, regardless of the specific area (voice, fluency, articulation, language, swallowing, etc.), are used because there is at least some research evidence that shows these techniques are effective. In cases where research evidence is lacking, we should at least be able to provide a theoretical justification for what we decide to do in treatment. This is where the two components of your graduate program, academic and clinical, come together. In your academic training, you will gain the foundational knowledge of each disorder, which includes, but is not limited to, theoretical bases for communication disorders, assessment protocols, and various treatment techniques. You will also become familiar with the research that backs it up. Once you have knowledge of the nature of disorders and assessment/treatment techniques that have been proven effective by research, you can begin to apply it to your clinical preparation (Figure 5–2). Based on the previous definition of EBP, it only makes sense that you would use this information in planning your treatment, regardless of the setting to which you are assigned for practicum. If you have considered your rationale for each goal and activity, you will be ready to explain why you

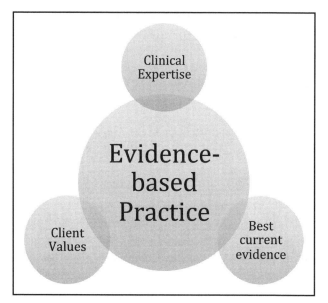

Figure 5–2. Evidence-based practice.

are choosing to work on certain targets. You want to be ready with your answer when your client, their caregivers, or other colleagues inquire about aspects of your treatment plan.

WHAT IS DATA?

You can have the perfect session planned with regard to activities and reinforcement but if you do not take the time to collect data, you have missed the boat. Although you may perceive that your client's articulation is better, data collected during your session will substantiate your opinion. When communicating with the client, his or her family, and other professionals, your data will be the objective foundation on which you base your recommendations. Not only should you gather data during each trial of the target behavior but you want to ensure that your data are accurate. Accurate data collection is essential to you providing competent services to your clients. Olswang and Bain (1994, p. 58) stress the importance of data in making accurate clinical decisions and note that data collection involves three preliminary steps, including making the decision of what to measure, how to measure, and how frequently to measure. Careful thought should be given to these steps, in that well-documented data should answer questions including what is effective in therapy, what needs to be modified, and when your client is meeting their goals.

Olswang and Bain (1994, p. 57) identify three principles that are paramount for data and methods of collection. These include that the data must be valid, reliable, and "collected in a reasonable fashion." As long as you are collecting data in a consistent manner, you may format your data sheet in any way you would like. Depending on the client's disorder and target behaviors, you may have a different format for each client. When deciding how to structure your session, it will be helpful to think about what you are taking data on, the cues, and the criteria. You should make every effort to take data during the session, however, the target behavior or individual client needs may preclude this. We have included several examples of data sheets in Appendix R for your reference. Data is usually reported in your SOAP note or other places as dictated by the setting you are in at the time. However, your data sheet may or may not be included in the client record. Regardless, baseline data should be obtained the first time the objective is targeted to have a way to measure progress. Calculating progress or lack thereof with regard to your goals guides your decision of when to modify goals and cues to best serve your client and his or her level of functioning. A helpful tool in tracking progress is a long-term graph. Please refer to Appendix T for examples.

In addition, the implementation of cues or prompts should be documented. A cue is used to help the client achieve a more accurate production than they are capable of without your assistance. There are many different types of cues including verbal cues, full model cues, and tactile cues. Your initial decision of which types of cues to use varies according to the client's disorder and level of functioning. Analysis of the effectiveness of the cues as represented in data collection may lead to your cueing hierarchy being altered.

Maintaining consistent and accurate data is paramount to determining when to discharge clients and offering support for your recommendations. Hegde and Davis (2010, p. 290) consider a target behavior to be trained "when its production in conversational speech in natural settings is acceptable."

For example, Hegde and Davis (2010) recommend the following criteria:

- "minimum of 90% accuracy for phonemes and language structures in conversational speech"
- "at least 90–95% of utterances or of speaking time for normal voice characteristics"
- "disfluencies not to exceed 3–4% in conversation in extraclinical situations"

While these guidelines may be appropriate for most clients, your competence as a growing clinician may lead you to discharge your client prior to reaching this criteria.

All settings, no matter how disparate they might appear at first glance, require practitioners to state goals and objectives, and these statements are always in written form. The following sections are designed to illustrate how goals and objectives are similar yet slightly different across work/practicum settings.

THE UNIVERSITY CLINIC

Most of you will begin your practicum experience in a university clinic. It is for this reason that throughout this book, we include examples of what forms and reports might look like in this setting. In the university setting, your paperwork requirements are more than in any other practicum environment. As we said in an earlier chapter, the intensity of the university setting in making you state rationales, goals, and objectives and write detailed reports is a valuable learning experience. As a beginning clinician in the university clinic, you may be asked to write a rationale for each goal you develop, and even though you won't continue to do this, it is good practice when you are first starting out. It teaches you how to think about clinical work and enables you to explain your approaches in any amount of detail required. If you gain experience writing behavioral objectives from scratch in the university clinic, you will have a lot less trouble dealing with the check boxes on a form in a medical setting or using a goal bank in a school system. Again, the important thing is the thought process and understanding *why* you choose to work on certain goals as a pathway to helping your client.

With the guidance of clinical supervisors you will find that the university clinic is an excellent setting in which you can learn the "ins and outs" of becoming a competent speech-language clinician. Because a university clinic traditionally operates on a semester by semester basis, your long-term and short-term goals are influenced by this time frame. You may find, however, that long-term goals do not vary much among settings. This is due to the fact that a long-term goal is not usually determined by a specific amount of time (unless in certain medical facilities). It is helpful to remember that a long-term goal is the ultimate change that you want to occur, and it is not always clear as to how long this will take or even if it will ultimately be achieved. What will vary, however, are your short-term goals and how they are written. We now examine what long-term and short-term goals might look like in the university clinic.

The Integration of Long-Term Goals (LTG), Short-Term Objectives (STO), and Rationales

Because you will see a number of different disorders across the life span in the university clinic, goals may be written many different ways. As mentioned previously, using the ABCD formula may be helpful when writing objectives, even when the objective is written in a simple sentence. Below you will find examples of long-term goals with a short-term objective (STO) and a rationale for each goal.

Client 1: 3-year-old male

Diagnosis: Limited expressive lexicon, normal receptive vocabulary, only uses single-word utterances (MLU 1.0).

LTG 1: The client will improve expressive language skills to an age-appropriate level in order to express wants and needs.

STO 1: (A) The client (B) will increase his expressive lexicon size to 75 (C) in spontaneous and imitative naming (D) at home and in clinical sessions as measured by sampling and parent reporting on a lexicon checklist.

Rationale: Two-word utterances are typically not produced by normally developing children until the lexicon size exceeds 50 (Nelson, 1973).

STO 2: (A) The client (B) will increase MLU to 2.0 (C) in spontaneous and imitative samples (D) taken at 2-week intervals during the semester, at home, and in the university clinical setting.

Rationale: Brown's stages of language development (Brown, 1973) indicate that a 3-year-old child should have a MLU of 2.5 to 3.9.

STO 3: (A) The client (B) will increase production of the basic operations of reference (nomination + X, recurrence + X, and nonexistence + X), (C) in spontaneous and imitative samples, (D) taken at 2-week intervals during the semester, at home and in the university clinical setting.

Rationale: Brown (1973) reported that the first types of word combinations seen in normal development are the basic operations of reference.

STO 4: (A) The client (B) will increase the production of the two-term semantic relations of agent + action and action + object, (C) in spontaneous and imitative samples, (D) taken at 2-week intervals during the semester at home and in the university clinical setting.

Rationale: Brown (1973) reported that agent + action and action + object are early developing semantic relations and they are the basis for SVO constructions.

Client 2: 22-year-old female

Diagnosis: Bilateral vocal nodules

LTG 1: The client will improve voice quality by reducing hoarseness in conversational speech using the facilitative technique of Anterior Focus.

STO: (A) The client (B) will reduce hoarseness using Anterior Focus (C) at the imitative phrase level while reading (D) as measured by a subjective voice quality rating scale administered by the clinician.

Rationale: Anterior or forward focus of the voice results in less abuse of the vocal folds and improved resonance (Boone, McFarlane, Von Berg, & Zraick, 2010).

Client 3: 5-year-old female

Diagnosis: Articulation disorder

LTG 1: The client will produce age-appropriate phonemes in all positions in conversation with 90% accuracy.

STO 1: The client will produce /k/ initial in words following the clinician's model with a visual stimulus with 90% accuracy.

STO 2: The client will produce /k/ final in words following the clinician's model with a visual stimulus with 90% accuracy.

STO 3: The client will produce /k/ medial in words following the clinician's model with a visual stimulus with 90% accuracy.

Rationale: According to Smit et al. (1990), 90% of females have acquired /k/ by the time they are 3 years, 6 months old; /k/ is an early developing phoneme.

Client 4: 22-year-old male

Diagnosis: Fluency disorder

LTG 1: The client will utilize appropriate fluency shaping techniques and strategies to increase verbal fluency in academic and social settings.

STO: The client will use Easy Onset while reading 3–4 word phrases in 8 out of 10 trials.

Rationale: Many people who stutter have difficulty on the initial word in an utterance; the Easy Onset or Easy Relaxed Approach (ERA) technique has proven very effective in initiating speech (Gregory, 2002).

Client 5: 33-year-old male

Diagnosis: English as a second language (ESL); difficulty with pronunciation of English phonemes.

LTG 1: The client will improve his use of Standard American English (SAE) in order to communicate more effectively in vocational and social settings.

STO 1: The client will correctly discriminate between minimal pairs /b/ and /v/ in words when provided with auditory stimuli for 90% accuracy.

STO 2: The client will correctly produce /v/ initial in words while reading from a word list with 90% accuracy.

Rationale: Van Riper and Emerick (1984) recommend that discrimination training occur prior to production training during the establishment phase of treatment; in addition, Locke (1980) states that only error sounds should be included in speech sound discrimination training.

Appendix H shows an example of a university clinic treatment plan.

MEDICAL SETTINGS

Setting goals in medical facilities is somewhat different from that in the university clinic, mainly due to the requirements of health care providers and insurance companies, or third-party payers. Any patient who receives speech therapy services in a medical facility will more than likely be covered by an insurance plan or plans (if he has private insurance in addition to Medicare or Medicaid). According to consumer-driven health care (CDHC), a third-party payment can be defined as "an insurer paying providers directly for services rendered to the insured, as opposed to an indemnity contract which pays the insured person for losses incurred" (CDHC, n.d.).

All health care facilities in the United States are governed by federal laws that regulate how payments are made, the codes used for billing, and the amount of time a patient can receive services. The Centers for Medicare and Medicaid Services (CMS) have the most updated information on Medicare billing procedures and regulations. You can find them on the Internet at http://www.cms.hhs.gov.

When requesting payment from a third-party payer for speech therapy services, the speech-language pathologist has to enter a billing code that corresponds with the patient's diagnosis and/or treatment. Diagnosis codes are published by the World Health Organization and are known as ICD-9-CM codes. This stands for International Classification of Diseases-9th revision (Clinical Modification).You will most likely hear them referred to as ICD-9 codes. Billing codes for treatment, also known as CPT or current procedural terminology codes, are published by the American Medical Association and are used in conjunction with ICD-9 codes. CPT codes, originally intended for physicians, are now used widely by many other practitioners (e.g., SLP, physical therapy, occupational therapy). All clinical documentation in a medical facility must support the codes that are billed. This also determines to some extent how goals are written and carried out in a medical setting.

As is the case in the university clinic, the SLP will first decide on a long-term goal for a patient in a medical facility; however, this is not true for all medical facilities. Some hospitals do not establish long-term goals, simply because a short-term goal is more efficacious. A hospital patient may be in an acute care unit for just a few days. In this case, a long-term goal is not necessary. For rehabilitation hospitals, the patient may only remain in a rehabilitation hospital for 7 to 21 days so long-term goals are written accordingly.

In writing a long-term goal for a patient in any type of medical facility, several factors must be taken into consideration. The SLP usually writes a long-term goal as a first step in establishing a *plan of care* (POC); however, there must be a written order from a physician requesting an evaluation and treatment for speech. For Medicare patients, the plan of care must not only be established and certified by a physician before treatment begins, it must be recertified by the physician every 30 or 60 days, depending on the setting (Paul, 1994).

In the following section, we provide examples of long-term goals as they would be written in a rehabilitation facility, hospital, and extended care setting. Keep in mind that in most medical facilities, there is often a "menu" of long-term goals listed,

and the SLP will simply check the appropriate goal; however, as a clinical practicum student, you will be expected to discern which goals will be appropriate for your patients based on the evaluation report.

Rehabilitation Setting

Often, in this setting, speech therapy (ST) notes are written on the same page with occupational therapy (OT) and/or physical therapy (PT) notes. At one of the sites that we visited, therapists from all three disciplines wrote their notes on one form. The areas to be targeted along with the patient's current level of functioning in each area were also listed. This provides a template for the therapist to go by when working with the patient. For example:

Communication/Cognitive

Parameter	Functional Level
Comprehension	Minimal (4)
Expression	Moderate (3)
Memory	Minimal (4)
Attention	Moderate (3)
Problem Solving	Moderate (3)
Swallowing	Independent (7)
Social Interaction	Supervision (5)

As you can see, charting like this is very minimal, and once the SLP fills in the appropriate information, it is used to work from each time he treats a patient. It is assumed that a patient who needs moderate assistance will be targeting the next higher level of independence (minimal assistance) as therapy progresses. The functional levels on the above chart are based on *functional independence measures*, or FIM scores, which are widely used in rehabilitation settings. These were developed by the Uniform Data System for Medical Rehabilitation at the State University of New York at Buffalo. You should know that *functional* is the operative word when writing speech and language goals for any patient, but especially so in the medical setting. To that end, *activities of daily living* (ADLs) are often mentioned in patient goals. At this point it is useful to provide a brief summary of FIM scores that you might see in medical treatment goals. The FIMs are used in medical facilities to gauge initial status of the patient and document progress in areas such as self care, bowel/bladder control, mobility, locomotion, communication, psychosocial adjustment, and cognitive function. These areas are rated using a seven-point scale that relates to the levels of assistance required by the patient to perform tasks (Frymark, 2003). The following are areas for which the speech-language pathologist may be responsible for scoring. Other disciplines such as nursing, physical therapy, and occupational therapy have their respective areas to score but may score these same areas as well.

7—Complete independence (timely, safely)

6—Modified independence (extra time, devices)

5—Supervision (cueing, setup)

4—Minimal assist (performs 75% or more of task)

3—Moderate assist (performs 50 to 74% of task)

2—Maximal assist (performs 25 to 49% of task)

1—Total assist (performs less than 25% of task)

Accurate FIM scores are vital as they guide the decision of the third-party payer as to how many days the patient may remain at the rehabilitation facility. Below you will find a sampling of some long-term goals from a rehabilitation facility. Note that the goals are concise. We also provide several examples of one short-term goal that might accompany these long-term goals. In addition to the following, a level of assistance may be specified after the goal.

Sample Long-Term Goals

At first glance, these goals may seem incomplete, confusing, or rather like a foreign language. Once you see them every day, however, they will begin to make sense and soon will become a regular part of your vocabulary.

- Express basic wants/needs via single words/ phrases/gestures/augmentative communication
- Identify and solve basic problems related to ADLs/vocational needs

- Follow simple directions (with or without cues) for ADLs
- Speak intelligibly to caregivers at word/phrase level
- Comprehend reading for paragraph length material
- Maximize verbal expression to clearly express complex thoughts/needs
- Perform oral-motor exercise program independently to maximize strength and ROM of oral musculature for speech/swallowing
- Yes/no reliability to facilitate care
- Write for ADLs (i.e., notes, checks)

As is evident from this list of goals, one of the most important factors in establishing long-term goals for patients in a medical facility is that the patient will be able to resume, to the greatest degree possible, their premorbid lifestyle. Most likely, the goal will be written in an abbreviated form [e.g., ↑ verbal expression and problem solving from MAX (2) to MOD (3),] with the "up arrow" meaning increase or improve. In the following examples, FIM scores are in parentheses after the corresponding level of assistance required.

LTG: Express basic wants and needs via single words or phrases independently.

STO: Patient will increase (↑) verbal expression for common object identification from MOD (3) to MIN (4).

LTG: Identify and solve basic problems related to ADLs/vocational needs with minimum assistance.

STO: Pt will ↑ verbal reasoning and problem solving from Total (1) to MAX (2).

LTG: Follow simple 1-step commands with supervision to increase independence with ADLs.

STO: Pt. will ↑ comprehension for simple 1-step commands from MOD (3) to MIN (4).

LTG: Speech intelligible to caregivers at word/ phrase level with MIN (4) assistance.

STO: Pt. will ↑ intelligibility at phrase level from MAX (2) to MOD (3).

LTG: Reading comprehension for functional material with MOD (3) assistance.

STO: Pt. will ↑ reading comprehension at the sentence level with MOD (3).

LTG: Utilize any means possible to communicate needs/wants independently.

STO: Pt. will perform functional object use with MAX (2).

LTG: Perform oral motor exercise program independently to maximize strength and ROM of oral musculature for speech/swallowing.

STO: Pt. will ↑ completion of OMEs from MIN (4) to SPV (5).

LTG: Increase yes/no reliability to facilitate care to MIN (4).

STO: Pt. will answer simple yes/no questions with MOD (3).

LTG: Perform functional written language tasks with supervision (5).

STO: Pt. will ↑ written expression for content of checks from MAX-2 to MOD-3.

Hospital Setting

As mentioned previously, the SLP in an acute care setting, such as in a hospital, may not develop long-term goals for patients, simply because the duration of their stay does not warrant them. In this case, the SLP will write one or more short-term goals for the patient, based on the initial evaluation. There will more than likely be a description of the patient's deficits included in the evaluation report, and it will be the job of the SLP to develop short-term goals based on this information. The short-term goals will be very similar to the ones listed above or may also be chosen from a menu of goals on a preprinted form. Often, abbreviations will be used instead of words. Refer to Appendix K for a partial list of common medical abbreviations, but keep in mind that these abbreviations may vary by state and facility.

Below is an example of short-term goals for patients in a hospital setting:

Patient 1: 72-year-old male

Primary diagnosis: Aphasia

STO 1: Increase (↑) auditory comprehension of one-step commands to 80% accuracy.

STO 2: Increase auditory comprehension of simple yes/no questions to 80% accuracy.

STO 3: Increase automatic speech to 80% accuracy.

Patient 2: 36-year-old male

Primary diagnosis: TBI

STO 1: Oriented to place and time of day with visual cues with 100% accuracy.

STO 2: Provide biographical information verbally when prompted with 80% accuracy.

STO 3: State solution to verbal problem solving situations related to ADLs in 10/12 trials.

Patient 3: 80-year-old female

Primary diagnosis: Dysarthria

STO 1: Pt will reduce nasal airflow by exaggerating oral movements while reading single words from a list independently in 8 out of 10 trials.

STO 2: ↑ speech intelligibility at phrase level to MIN-4.

Note that abbreviations are often used in a hospital setting, as well. In these examples, OME stands for *oral motor exercises* and an up arrow indicates "improve" or "increase."

Patients usually do not remain in an acute care setting for an extended period of time, and your goal, if you are the SLP who is treating this patient, is to figure out what will be most beneficial to this patient during his stay in acute care. This is based on information collected during the patient's evaluation, input from the family (when available), and the patient's prognosis. Refer to Appendix I for more examples of goal writing in a rehab hospital setting.

Long-Term Care/Nursing Home

Long-term care (LTC), *extended care, skilled nursing facility* (frequently referred to as SNF), and *nursing home* are names that apply to a facility that provides a range of health, personal care, social, and housing services to people who are unable to care for themselves independently. The SLP who works in one of these facilities will perform many of the same services as an SLP in a hospital or rehabilitation setting; the main difference is the duration of services provided, and this is determined in large part by Medicare.

Any student who has a practicum experience in a LTC facility will become familiar with Medicare, and the terms *Part A* and *Part B*. For the purpose defined in this text, you will not need to have a detailed knowledge of Medicare and its components; however, it is important to know that patients are billed either under Part A or Part B, depending on their age, diagnosis, and length of stay in the facility. Patients who are considered *acute* and are receiving skilled nursing, usually in the first 100 days following their move from the hospital to the LTC facility, are billed under Part A. Patients who are considered more *chronic* and have been in the LTC facility for more than 100 days are billed under Part B (i.e., a patient suddenly begins having difficulty swallowing and is referred to the SLP for evaluation and treatment, even though he has been in the LTC facility for 8 months).

Another reason we mention Part A and Part B in this section is that the requirement for progress notes is different for each one: for Part A, the SLP will complete a weekly note, and for Part B he will complete a daily note. Because most patients in a LTC facility are covered by Medicare, this billing system is the driving force behind how therapy is carried out as well as how all of the supporting paperwork is completed.

Let's examine what goals may look like in a long-term care or nursing home setting. Some LTC facilities provide a "goal bank" for long-term and short-term goals. The following are some examples of long-term goals.

Long-term goals may include:

- Patient will improve the ability to adequately self-monitor swallowing skills and perform appropriate compensatory techniques independently.
- Patient will facilitate safe swallowing skills with least restrictive diet via use of compensatory strategies, diet modifications, and caregiver/family education with 90% accuracy.
- The patient will effectively communicate basic wants/needs with 100% accuracy with no cues.
- The patient will tolerate highest possible diet with the use of compensatory strategies 100% of the time without signs/symptoms of aspiration to optimize nutrition and hydration.
- The patient will improve cognitive function including attention skills to independent, memory skills to supervision and problem-solving abilities to supervision to allow for increase functional integration into environment and complete activities of daily living.

Short-term goals may include:

- The patient will name objects, pictures, people, and/or activities independently in order to improve verbalizations.
- The patient will perform verbal sentence completion tasks increasing to minimal level of impairment given 5% verbal instruction/cues to increase automatic verbalizations.
- The patient will communicate/verbalize mental awareness of person, place, and time (×3) given 50% verbal instruction/cues in order to increase functional integration into environment.
- The patient will improve safety awareness for self care tasks with minimal assistance (1–25% assist).

Although goals in a LTC setting may not always be written in this way, two things are usually true regarding goals for patients in a medical setting: (a) they are meant to be functional and (b) they are written in order to restore the patient, to the greatest extent possible, to his prior level of functioning.

SCHOOL SETTING

Any student who completes a speech pathology clinical practicum in the public schools will encounter the *Individualized Education Program*, or IEP. For any students who have an opportunity to serve children ages birth to 3 years, whether in a preschool, Head Start, or Early Intervention program, the *Individualized Family Services Plan*, or IFSP, will also become familiar. In order for you to understand treatment planning and goal setting in the public school environment, we need to provide some background. It is important for you to know that school systems operate the way they do not because of arbitrary decisions made by school districts, but due to the existence of many complex layers of federal and state law.

Individualized Education Program (IEP)

The IEP is a written plan outlining the special education program and/or other services (speech therapy) required by a particular student. It identifies learning expectations that are modified from or alternative to the expectations for the appropriate grade and subject, including measurable goals and benchmarks for each goal. It also identifies any accommodations or modifications needed to assist the student in achieving his learning expectations. In addition, the IEP provides a framework for monitoring and reporting progress to parents.

Every student who has been identified as eligible for special education services of any kind must have an IEP. This applies to students who receive speech therapy as a part of other special education services, as well as to students who are served through the general education curriculum and are pulled out for speech therapy.

To create an effective IEP, parents, teachers, administrators, other related services personnel, and sometimes even the student must come together to determine unique needs. These individuals must design an educational program that will help the student be involved in the general curriculum to the greatest extent possible and make educational progress.

The Individuals with Disabilities Education Act (IDEA) requires certain information to be included in each child's IEP; however, states and local school systems often include additional information in IEPs in order to meet federal or state laws. The flexibility that states and school systems have to design their own IEP forms is one reason why IEP forms may look different across school systems or states (United States Department of Education [DOE], 2008).

No Child Left Behind (NCLB) was passed on January 8, 2002, and also impacted the operation of school systems. NCLB is built on four principles: (a) accountability for results, (b) more choices for parents, (c) greater local control and flexibility, and (d) an emphasis on doing what works based on scientific research. We do not entertain a detailed discussion regarding NCLB in this book; however, we state that due to the realignment of IDEA with NCLB, there now are certain guidelines that all school systems must follow regarding the IEP.

The IEP Development Process

As mentioned previously, the IEP is a written description of an appropriate instructional program for a student with special needs. In order to understand IEP goals, it is useful to know how an IEP is generated. One major difference is that the IEP is developed by a multidisciplinary team of professionals, so the SLP is not writing goals in a vacuum. There are six steps that must be followed in the process of establishing an IEP for any student:

1. **Prereferral:** This is an informal process that involves the classroom teacher identifying the student's educational problems and suggesting solutions. These interventions are attempted for a 6-week period.
2. **Referral:** If the interventions put in place during the prereferral are not successful, then a referral to special education is made. It should be noted that only those students with academic performance extensively behind that of their

classmates and/or those who exhibit learning, emotional, and behavioral difficulties can be officially referred. Once the referral is made, an IEP team is created. This team consists of the student's parent(s)/guardian, special education teacher, one general education teacher, and any other professionals who may need to provide services to the student.

3. **Evaluation:** Once the referral has been made, the student must be evaluated to determine if a disability exists, whether special education is required, and, if so, what types of special or related services are needed. The type of evaluation that is performed will be based on the deficits identified during the prereferral and referral processes. Tests may be administered to assess learning, communication, behavior, or a combination of modalities. Federal law mandates that the IEP team must use at least two formal assessments, and that these assessments take place in the student's native language in order to make a determination of eligibility for special education. The team has 60 days from the referral date to determine eligibility.

4. **Eligibility:** Once the results of the evaluation are prepared, the IEP team will meet to determine if the student meets eligibility requirements. There must be a unanimous decision by the team for the student to be referred for special education services.

5. **Development of an IEP:** Following eligibility determination, the team will decide on the appropriate services and placement for the student, preferably in the least restrictive environment (LRE). A broad definition of LRE is an educational setting where a child with disabilities can receive a free appropriate education designed to meet his or her needs while being educated with peers without disabilities in the regular education environment to the maximum extent appropriate. It is during this phase of IEP development that specific goals are generated. We discuss this specifically in the next section.

6. **Annual Review:** The IEP team is responsible for conducting an annual review to ensure that the student is meeting goals and/or making progress on the benchmarks specified for each

objective that was developed by the team. This review takes place on a yearly basis; however, if the IEP needs to be modified or otherwise updated, a meeting may be called at any time, by any member of the IEP team, to make these revisions.

Components of the IEP

Now that we have discussed the steps involved in creating the IEP, we outline the specific components, along with the purpose for each. One thing that is important to keep in mind regarding IEPs is that even though they must contain the same basic information, the format may look different from state to state. In researching information from various regions across the country, we found that many states provide copies of their IEP forms on the state's department of education Web site. What we also found is that, with a few exceptions, most of the forms follow roughly the same format. Thus, although the IEP format will vary within and across states, there are standard criteria that must be included, regardless of where the document is being written. The IEP contains the following basic components:

- **Student Profile/Present Level of Educational Performance (PLEP):** This section outlines biographical data on the student, how the student is performing academically, and a description of the student's speech and/or language deficits.
- **Progress Reporting:** The IEP states how parents are to be informed of the student's progress, including frequency (at least as often as nondisabled students) and method, whether written reports, phone calls, or conferences.
- **Special Instructional Factors:** This section is for the purpose of identifying if the student has any limitations that will impede his learning, such as hearing or visual impairment, limited English proficiency, the need for assistive technology, or adaptive physical education.
- **Transition Services:** This section is designed to address the needs of students in high school in order to implement programs that will enable them to transition from school to a vocational setting or postsecondary education (the age

of transition varies from state to state, and can start as early as 14 years). Transition information must address the following areas: (a) recreation and leisure; (b) community participation; (c) postsecondary training and learning opportunities; (d) home living; and (e) work (job and job training).

■ **Transfer of Rights:** This section informs the parent/student that all rights pertaining to special education services transfer to the student at age 18 years. The date the student was notified of the transfer of rights must be indicated in this section of the IEP. Parents must be given a *Notice of Transfer of Parental Rights.*

■ **Goals:** These include broad statements that describe what a student can reasonably be expected to accomplish within a 12-month period of time in a special education program. Goals focus on skills or behaviors, must be related to the child's PLEP, and must be measurable. They must include the student's present level and expected level of performance.

■ **Benchmarks:** Also known as objectives, benchmarks are measurable, intermediate steps leading to the attainment of the goal. There must be at least two benchmarks per goal, and they must include the following: skill/behavior, conditions, criteria, and evaluation methods similar to our earlier discussion of behavioral objectives.

■ **Special Education and Related Services:** In this section you will find the type of service being provided (speech therapy) and the anticipated frequency, duration, location, and beginning and ending date of services. This section also includes, if necessary, supplementary aids and services, accommodations needed for assessments, assistive technology, and any other related services.

■ **Extended School Year (ESY):** The term *extended school year* encompasses a range of options in providing programs in excess of the traditional 180-day school year, due to issues of regression (loss of skills during an absence of intervention) and recoupment (recovering skills that were lost). In most cases, the IEP team will

meet to determine if a student is eligible for ESY and make the appropriate recommendations.

■ **Least Restrictive Environment (LRE):** Refers to the amount of time a student with a disability will participate in the regular classroom with nondisabled peers. An explanation of when and why the student will be excluded from the regular classroom is required.

■ **Signature Section:** The signature of everyone in attendance at the IEP meeting, or who will participate in carrying out the student's IEP, is found in this section. There are generally specific titles listed, such as parent, local educational agency (LEA) representative, special education teacher, general education teacher, student, and other agency representative. There is space for other names to be added, if necessary.

Individualized Family Services Plan (IFSP)

The IFSP came about as a result of *The Program for Infants and Toddlers with Disabilities,* or Part C of IDEA. Part C is a federal grant program that assists states in operating a comprehensive statewide program or early intervention services for infants and toddlers with disabilities, serving children from birth through age 3 years and their families. The program was originally established by Congress in 1986 in recognition of "an urgent and substantial need" to enhance the development of infants and toddlers with disabilities; reduce educational costs by minimizing the need for special education through early intervention; minimize the likelihood of institutionalization and maximize independent living; and enhance the capacity of families to meet their child's needs. Children served under Part C of IDEA are those with developmental delay "as measured by appropriate diagnostic instruments and procedures" including: (a) cognitive development; (b) physical development, including vision and hearing; (c) communication development; (d) social or emotional development, and (e) adaptive development (IDEA, 2004). An IFSP documents and guides the early intervention process for children with disabilities and their families. It is the vehicle through which effective early intervention is implemented in accordance with Part C of the IDEA. It contains information about the services necessary to facilitate a child's development and enhance the family's capacity to facilitate the child's development. Through this process, family members and service providers work as a team to plan, implement, and evaluate services tailored to the family's unique concerns, priorities, and resources (IDEA, 2004).

How Is the IFSP Different from the IEP?

There are several factors that distinguish the IEP from the IFSP, but the first and most noticeable difference is the inclusion of the word *family*. The name *Individualized Family Service Plan* was chosen because the family is the constant in a child's life and is therefore the focus of the intervention plan. According to the Council for Exceptional Children, there are several ways in which the IFSP differs from the IEP:

■ It includes outcomes targeted for the family, as opposed to focusing only on the eligible child.
■ It includes the notion of natural environments, which encompass home or community settings. This focus creates opportunities for learning interventions in everyday routines and activities, rather than only in formal, contrived environments.
■ It includes activities undertaken with multiple agencies beyond the scope of Part C (see explanation below). These are included to integrate all services into one plan.
■ It names a service coordinator to help the family during the development, implementation, and evaluation of the IFSP.

The family's concerns, priorities, and resources guide the entire IFSP process. Early intervention should be seen as a system of services and supports available to families to enhance their capacity to care for their children.

There are also several ways that the IFSP is similar to the IEP. As noted in the section on the IEP, you will find that an IFSP also has the following:

■ A statement of the child's present levels of development
■ A statement of the family's strengths and needs related to enhancing the child's development
■ A statement of major outcomes expected to be achieved for the child and family
■ The criteria, procedures, and time lines for determining progress
■ The specific early intervention services necessary to meet the unique needs of the child and the family, including the frequency, intensity, and method of delivery
■ The natural environment(s) in which services will be provided, including justification, if any, of why the services will not be provided in a natural environment
■ The projected dates for initiation of services and their anticipated duration
■ Name of the service provider who is responsible for implementing the plan and coordinating with other agencies
■ Steps to support the child's transition to preschool or other appropriate services

One thing that you can see from the above goals of the IFSP is the importance of goal setting. Note that it mentions specific objectives, ways to measure them, and who will measure progress. Appendix L provides an example of an IFSP.

How Does the IEP Reflect Specific Goals?

Any child who has an IEP will have specific annual goals and benchmarks to go along with those goals for every area in which he is receiving special education services, such as reading, math, language, and speech.

You may be asking yourself, what is an annual goal? What is a benchmark? These and other questions are answered in this section, as we explore the world of goal writing in the public schools.

We have been talking about long-term and short-term goals and up until this point have not mentioned anything about benchmarks. The reason for this is that the term *benchmark* is relative only to

IEP paperwork. To provide a brief definition, *benchmarks are major milestones that specify skill or performance levels a student needs to accomplish toward reaching his annual goal.* You might be thinking that this is similar to the definition of a short-term goal, and you are exactly correct. Depending on the state, either benchmarks or short-term goals or both are used interchangeably on the IEP. For example, according to the Nebraska Department of Education Web site, a benchmark represents the actual content or performance the student is to accomplish at a specific interval or grade level. It defines a short-term objective as a measurable, intermediate step between a student's present level of educational performance (PLEP) and the annual goals established for the student (Nebraska, 2006). In the state of New Mexico, the goals page is titled, "Annual Goals and Short-Term Objectives or Benchmarks." In Tennessee, the same page is titled, "Measurable Annual Goals and Benchmarks/Short-term Instructional Objectives for IEP/Transition Activities," and in California, the page is simply titled, "Annual Goals and Objectives." See Appendix M for an example of an IEP. Keep in mind that there are software programs that generate IEPs, and many school systems use these. Based on state requirements, school system policies, and how goals are written, you simply fill in the student's information, and the IEP will be generated for you.

Both benchmarks and short-term objectives are developed based on a logical breakdown of the annual goal and guide the development and modification, as necessary, of strategies that will be most effective in realizing the goals. Goals provide a system for measuring the student's progress toward long-range expectations. After the IEP team develops measurable goals for a student, it must develop effective strategies to realize those goals and measurable, intermediate steps (short-term objectives) or major milestones (benchmarks) that enable families, students, and educators to monitor progress.

Let's take a look at some examples of benchmarks:

1. The student will prepare verbal, written, and visual compositions that fulfill different purposes (to inform, to persuade, to narrate, to entertain).
2. The student will identify and use appropriate language in different settings (school, home, community).

3. The student will understand place value up to three-digit numbers.

Examples of short-term objectives include:

1. David will write answers to simple addition facts with sums 0 to 20 (4 + 5) in 5 minutes on a worksheet at a rate of 40 digits correct per minute with no errors by October 2013.
2. Given different board games and two to three peers, Mary will play cooperatively for 15 consecutive minutes for 10 turn-taking exchanges.

Below you will find some examples of annual goals and benchmarks from two different states. We will start with each student's present level of educational performance (PLEP) and then include annual goals and benchmarks to support the annual goal.

Student 1

PLEP: John exhibits difficulties putting his thoughts on paper. He is very creative but does not understand sentence construction or how to develop paragraphs. He needs to use punctuation and capitalization consistently. John received 12 out of 50 points on the district's assessment for expressive writing. He needs to learn to write the four different sentence types (simple, compound, complex, compound-complex) correctly and integrate them into a paragraph.

Measurable Annual Goal: In 36 weeks John will write at least a six-sentence paragraph using at least three different sentence types scoring 45/50 on the writing rubric.

Benchmarks:
1. John will write simple sentences.
2. John will write compound sentences.
3. John will write complex sentences.
4. John will write compound-complex sentences.

Student 2 (from a different state)

PLEP: David is a 4-year-old male who lives with his parents and two older brothers. He attends a preschool at his church three times per week. His teacher reports that he interacts well with his peers at preschool. She also indicated on a checklist that David is more difficult to understand than the other children in the class and does not use sentences as long as those of the other children. He has a history of ear infections and has had two sets of PE tubes placed in his ears. He is reported to also have trouble with allergies and infrequent episodes of asthma. Phoneme production deficits adversely affect phonological awareness and his limited expressive skills restrict his participation in oral classroom activities and social interaction in the preschool environment. Standardized testing revealed reduced vocabulary development and mean length of utterance (MLU). He cannot answer questions appropriately. His articulation errors are developmentally inappropriate for a child his age and cause his speech to be difficult to understand to both familiar and unfamiliar listeners. David becomes easily frustrated when not understood.

Measurable Annual Goal: By May 2013, David will verbally express himself by using four- to five-word sentences while asking/answering "wh" questions 8/10 trials in structured conversational analysis.

Benchmarks:

1. By the end of the first 9 weeks, David will answer "who" and "what" questions using stories and pictures as stimuli with 80% accuracy.

2. By the end of the second 9 weeks, David will answer "where" and "when" questions using stories and pictures as stimuli with 80% accuracy.

3. By the end of the third 9 weeks, David will ask "who" and "what" questions using books, pictures, and orally read stories as stimuli with 80% accuracy.

Measurable Annual Goal: David will eliminate use of final consonant deletion by producing the target phonemes /p,m,n,b,k,g,d,t/ in the final position with 90% accuracy in structured oral activities in his preschool classroom as measured by SLP progress monitoring.

Benchmarks:

1. By the end of the first 9 weeks, David will imitate the target phonemes at the word level with 80% accuracy.

2. By the end of the second 9 weeks, David will produce the target phonemes at the spontaneous word level with 80% accuracy.

3. By the end of the third 9 weeks, David will produce the target phonemes at the spontaneous phrase/sentence level with 80% accuracy.

4. By the end of the fourth 9 weeks, David will produce the target phonemes in structured oral activities with 90% accuracy.

As you can see, goals, benchmarks, and objectives are written quite differently across states, and it will be up to you to familiarize yourself with your school's process. What is also important to consider is that goals, benchmarks, and objectives must be written so they can pass the "stranger test." In other words, they should be written so that someone who did not write them could use them to develop appropriate instructional plans and assess student progress. They should also be written to pass the "so what test," meaning the IEP team considers the importance of the goal, objective, or benchmark. The team would pose the question, "Is the skill indicated in this goal, objective, or benchmark really an important skill for the student to learn?" If the answer is "No," then most likely, the goal isn't appropriate. In many ways, this is similar to the functional goals targeted in medical environments with adults. For children, the ability to function in the school environment is an important aspect of their lives.

SIMILARITIES AND DIFFERENCES ACROSS WORK SETTINGS

Figure 5–3 illustrates goal writing similarities and differences across university, medical, and educational settings. We first remind you about similarities. First, every work setting requires that goals are set and that they are written down in some format. Second, the goals must be measurable and thus written to some degree as behavioral objectives. A third

Goal-Writing Differences Across Work Settings

University	Medical	School
• Not team oriented • Goals written in client folder • Goals may be functional • Goals longer and more descriptive • Procedures are more detailed • More extensive data gathered in samples • Rationale often provided • Goals can be changed quickly • Goals are for semester	• Team oriented • Goals written in patient chart • Goals must be functional • Behavioral • Objectives very brief with abbreviations • Smaller samples gathered • Use of FIM Scores • Wording of goals important for reimbursement • Rationale implied but not written • Goals often for short time periods	• Team oriented • Goals written on IEP • Goals educationally based • Goals written in medium length • Moderate sized samples • Rationale implied or loosely stated • Difficult to change goals without IEP meeting • Goals are annual with periodic benchmarks

Goal-Writing Similarities Across Work Settings

- Written goals are required
- Goals must be written behaviorally
- Periodic measurement is required to determine progress
- Documentation of progress is important
- Functional relevance of goals is optimal

Figure 5–3. Similarities and differences of goal writing across work settings.

similarity is that in all settings the SLP is required to take periodic measurements to determine if the client is making progress toward the goal that was initially set. Fourth, documentation is viewed as critical in all work settings. Finally, the functional relevance of goals is important in all work settings. While a student in a university clinic could write a goal that was not particularly functional, it is always ideal to develop goals that are functionally relevant. Obviously, in medical settings functional goals are mandated, and in educational settings, academic relevance is paramount.

Goal-setting differences across work settings revolve around several issues. First, there can be more or less involvement of multidisciplinary teams in developing goals. This is more important in medical and school settings than in the university clinic. The place where goals are written down is a second difference among settings. In the university setting, we write goals in treatment plans or reports that are placed in a client's folder. In medical settings, the goals are part of a patient's medical chart. In school systems, the IEP is the place to write goals. A third difference in goal writing is the length and form of the goal statements. In the university setting, goals are written in narrative form and tend to be lengthier than in other settings. In the medical setting, goals are brief and there is liberal use of medical abbreviations. Goals in school systems are often midway between university and medical settings in length. A fourth difference among settings is the length of the sample gathered to verify progress toward goals. In the university, it is not unusual for students to take language samples several times during a semester to verify progress. On the other hand, medical settings use short tasks and FIM scores to monitor patient progress. School systems, again, are midway between medical settings and university clinics. They often monitor progress with nonstandardized tasks but also give standardized assessments on an annual basis to see if change has occurred. A fifth difference among settings is the presence of a written rationale for goals. In the university setting, students are given practice in developing rationales as part of their goals when they are first beginning practicum. Rationales are almost never seen in the documentation produced by medical facilities and school systems. A sixth difference among settings is the ability to easily change goals. In medical facilities the use of reimbursement codes and oversight by the medical establishment may make it difficult to change goals quickly. In the school setting it may require the IEP team to reconvene to discuss changes in objectives. The university clinic can change goals whenever the practicum supervisor feels it is necessary.

It is also important to mention computerized reports again in this section. Not only do software programs generate diagnostic reports; they can also create progress reports, treatment plans, and discharge notes. Depending on the facility, you may find that you are writing reports on your own or that all you do is enter the client data into a computer and the report is generated for you. Either way, you still have to discern what information is pertinent and where to write it. It is our hope that the information in this book is helpful and that you will gain this valuable insight through your clinical practicum experiences. Our discussion of goal writing has attempted to introduce the practicum student to the elements of well-crafted goals that apply to any work environment. We have also tried to alert students to the changes in goal writing that will be encountered as they do clinical practicum across different types of settings. Goal writing at each facility will be tailored to the client's specific needs, whether they are focused on academic needs or needs they encounter every day (functional). Hopefully, you will take some comfort in the similarities and view the differences as a challenge and not a threat.

6 Short-Term Progress Reporting

> **Supervisor in medical facility:** "I'm having a hard time understanding what you wrote here about your therapy session. What do all of these numbers mean?"
>
> **Student:** "Well, uh . . . I tried to write down my data so that it makes sense. Why is this so important, anyway? I know he's making progress—isn't that all that matters?"
>
> **Supervisor:** "Of course it matters that he's making progress, but you need to have the right documentation to back it up, especially if we want to get paid!"

Ah, the real world . . . the place where money is the name of the game—at least, that is, if you're talking about the real world of hospitals, nursing homes, or a private practice. Here, billing policies, copayments, insurance claims, and reimbursement are an everyday part of life. Patients must pay for services, and in most cases, their health insurance, whether it's Medicare, Medicaid, or private, will cover the cost.

There are places, however, where this is not the case. Take for instance, the public schools. There, you don't have to worry about establishing fees for your services, filing insurance claims, or methods of payment. And unless you work in a school system that bills Medicaid, you don't have to worry about payments for services at all.

Yes, it is true that in many parts of the real world, you won't get paid if you don't have the adequate documentation to back up what you're doing in therapy. But it's also true that even in the world of the university clinic, which some will claim is not "the real world," you learn to report on your clients' progress because it is an integral part of the therapy process—not just because you won't get paid! You would think a doctor was crazy if he put you on medication for an infection and then commented, "Well, we just thought we'd try those pills for the heck of it. We don't really care what effect they're having." Reporting on the progress of your clients and/or patients is paramount to a successful course of treatment. According to Paul (1994), "Clear and comprehensive records are necessary to justify the need for treatment, to document the effectiveness of that treatment, and to have a legal record of events." In addition, as cited in Middleton et al. (2001, p. 39), the ASHA Professional Services Board (ASHA, 1990), which defines standards for clinical service in speech-language pathology, states, "The quality of services provided is evaluated and documented on a systematic and continuing basis." In other words, the only way for you to know if what you are doing in therapy is working is to take accurate data, analyze that data on a daily or weekly basis, and then make modifications accordingly. Otherwise, you are just "tilting at windmills," as the saying goes.

At this point, you may be asking yourself, "But how will I know how to do this?" For starters, one of the main purposes of this book is to expose you to the paperwork and reporting requirements you will be expected to master by the time you finish your graduate work. That way, when you are called upon to complete any type of reporting function, whether it's related to assessment or treatment, you will at least have an idea of what to expect. In addition, your clinical supervisor(s) will assist you a great deal when you begin your clinical practicum experience. ASHA understands the importance of good supervision when it relates to students in training—so much so, in fact, that it has outlined 13 supervisory "tasks" that inform student clinicians of what to expect from their supervisors. These guidelines insure that all students enrolled in SLP practicum will be guided and directed in all areas of service delivery by a competent, licensed clinician.

DAILY PROGRESS REPORTING

There would be no way to measure the efficacy of your speech-language therapy if not for daily progress reporting. Data that taken during each therapy session is used to determine several things: (a) if the patient/client is making progress, (b) that the treatment techniques are appropriate, (c) when modifications need to be made, and (d) how to plan for future sessions.

The SOAP note, as it's affectionately known in the world of SLP, is a staple of daily reporting on client progress. *SOAP* is an acronym that stands for *subjective*, *objective*, *assessment*, and *plan*. SOAP notes are also commonly used by medical and rehabilitation staff and therefore may appear frequently in other sections of medical charts.

The following is a description of each area of the SOAP note and an example of the information contained therein:

Subjective (S): A description of the client's physical and/or emotional state, including affect, mood, level of motivation, attention, and so on. It is also appropriate to report relevant client or family comments.

"S" Example 1: Mr. Jones was in a pleasant mood during therapy today, although he stated that he was a little tired. His wife said, "He didn't sleep well last night" and he reported difficulty concentrating during the session.

"S" Example 2: Cowan was eager to begin therapy today. She told the clinician, "I've been practicing my new /s/ sound!"

Objective (O): Includes information regarding the target behaviors, session goals and data for each goal. If testing was done, write the name of the test(s) administered and the results. According to Moon-Meyer (2004), *the facts* belong in the objective part of the SOAP note. In addition to your data, you want to include any information that will support a statement made in the subjective part (Moon-Meyer, 2004).

"O" Example 1: The client will improve immediate memory by using chunking to recall six digit sequences with 75% accuracy.

Data: Mr. Jones achieved 4/10 = 40% correct responses on his first attempt. When he was reinstructed with regard to the technique of chunking and the stimuli was repeated, performance increased to 8/10 = 80% accuracy.

"O" Example 2: The client will produce /s/ final imitatively in phrases modeled by the clinician while playing a board game with 80% accuracy.

Data: Cowan achieved 17/20 (85%) accuracy today. Cue 2 increased accuracy to 100%.

Assessment (A): Includes an explanation of what your data means and factors that may have affected performance. Also includes a note about the type of stimuli, if necessary, and the effectiveness of cues and reinforcement.

"A" Example 1: Mr. Jones's accuracy was decreased from previous sessions due to reported fatigue and lack of concentration. Repeating the stimulus and a verbal cue to chunk the information increased his accuracy significantly.

"A" Example 2: Cowan met criteria for the third consecutive week when using the same stimuli to target /s/ initial phrases. Cue 2 (use of a mirror) was effective when cues were needed.

Plan (P): Includes a statement about what is planned for the next treatment session and a rationale for why. May include reference to goals, cues, reinforcement, and stimuli.

"P" Example 1: Mr. Jones was given homework to practice with his wife. Chunking will continue to be targeted and if difficulty persists, a written prompt may be provided. Cues should remain the same due to effectiveness.

"P" Example 2: Increase goal to /s/ initial spontaneous phrases while playing "Fish-n-Say." Use probe list to assess generalization to other positions. Restructure cues based on goal modification. Continue reinforcement with stickers due to Cowan's increased motivation.

Now that we know what is contained in the SOAP note, let's examine what one will look like across the various settings and how they are used in everyday treatment.

UNIVERSITY CLINIC

As a practicum student in the university clinic, you will serve clients with a variety of diagnoses across the life span. In almost all university clinics, students are taught to use the SOAP note as the primary tool for data reporting. In our clinic, students write a SOAP note for each session, whether the client comes one, two, or three times per week. This may not be the case in all clinics. In other situations, students may write just one note for the week, regardless of how many sessions are included. It should be noted that the SOAP note should be concise and detailed, although abbreviations can be used, and information does not have to be communicated using complete sentences as long as it is understandable to the person reading the note.

In our clinic, every client has a confidential file that is kept in a locked cabinet in our clinic office. For each speech client, there is an additional "working file," in a secure location where daily therapy plans and SOAP notes are filed, along with a record of the student's clinical hours.

In some settings, speech-language pathologists (SLPs) fill out weekly and monthly progress reports; however, this is not usually the case in the university clinic. In general, the SOAP notes are used to record all of the data for the semester, and then this information is summarized in the end of semester treatment or progress report. For this reason, information contained in the SOAP note must be timely and accurate. Without accurate data, it is very difficult to determine if true progress is being made. Let's examine a few SOAP notes from clients in the university clinic.

Example 1: Aphasia Client

Subjective: Mr. Smith was pleasant and cooperative today. He put forth good effort throughout the session, except with confrontational naming, which seemed to frustrate him.

Objective:

STO 1: The client will spontaneously match a picture to a corresponding written phrase description from a field of 3 with 70% accuracy.

Data: 11/15 = 73%; increased to 13/15 = 87% with elimination cue

STO 2: The client will spontaneously name common household objects with 60% accuracy.

Data: 4/12 = 33%; cues did not increase accuracy

STO 3: The client will provide the missing word in a common phrase with minimal cues from the clinician with 80% accuracy.

Data: 3/10 = 30% with minimal cueing; increased to 70% with phonemic cue

STO 4: The client will copy the clinician's written model of personal/pertinent information with 100% accuracy.

Data: 5/5 = 100%

Assessment: Mr. Smith's reading comprehension improved from last session; however, he continues to exhibit significant anomia during verbal structured and unstructured tasks. He had a particularly difficult time with confrontational naming today and abandoned the attempt quickly. He required increased time to respond to the phrase completion task, and needed frequent phonemic cues. Criteria has been met for copying personal information over the past three sessions; this goal will be modified to increase complexity of this task.

Plan: Continue to target expressive language skills and encourage use of gestures when pt. is unable to circumlocute for verbal communication. Modify goal of confrontational naming due to level of difficulty. Vary stimuli for reading comprehension task to assess generalization. Provide phonemic cue first in order to increase success with common phrases. Modify written language goal to target personal information with only a partial model and provide corresponding homework.

Example 2: Child Language Client

Subjective: Max was very active today, and required frequent redirection to attend. His mother stated, "He has a lot of energy this morning!"

Objective:

STO 1: The client will respond appropriately to "what" and "where" questions after listening to a 4- to 5-sentence story with 80% accuracy.
Data: 10/20 = 50%; increased to 75% with repeat of stimuli

STO 2: The client will identify the phoneme when provided with the sound for all short vowels with 100% accuracy.
Data: 7/10 = 70%; increased to 100% when given choice cue

STO 3: The client will read 10 out of 15 sight words when presented on flash cards by the clinician.
Data: 8/15

Assessment: Max's performance on "wh" questions decreased from previous sessions; however, this may be attributed to his high energy level and difficulty focusing. He enjoyed the Bingo game used during the vowel activity and his accuracy increased to 100% when given a choice cue, indicating improvement from the previous session. When in error, Max continues to identify /ɛ/ for /ɪ/. He exhibited hesitation recognizing sight words, although today was the first session these words were targeted. He tends to get easily distracted throughout the session, so he may benefit from more frequent breaks.

Plan: Continue to target "what" and "where" questions, using repetition when needed; a cue such as "make sure your listening ears are on" should be implemented prior to reading the story. Continue working on short vowels but introduce long vowels. The same sight words should be targeted to increase speed of identification and accuracy. Homework should be given for daily practice. Initiate use of schedule board and high interest reward to increase attention.

Example 3: Child Articulation Client

Subjective: Hannah was very happy today and ready to begin therapy. Hannah's mother reported that her teacher said she is understanding more of Hannah's speech.

Objective:

STO 1: The client will spontaneously produce /k/ in the initial position of words while naming picture cards with 80% accuracy.

Data: 2/12 = 17% with maximum cues

STO 2: The client will produce /f/ in the initial position of words while playing Articulation Bingo with 80% accuracy.

Data: 4/12 = 33%; increased to 8/12 = 67% with verbal cue and 10/12 = 83% with full model

Assessment: Hannah had significant difficulty producing /k/ initial in spontaneous words and continues to substitute /t/. She also substituted /t/ for /f/ initial; however, the verbal cue of "put your teeth on your lip" was beneficial. She responded well to stickers and was motivated by a schedule board.

Plan: Modify /k/ initial to imitative words to determine facilitating context and modify cueing hierarchy accordingly. Continue to use Bingo to target /f/, since Hannah enjoys the game and present phonetic placement as first cue. Provide Hannah's mom with education regarding phonetic placement so she can implement cueing at home. Continue with current reinforcement.

Example 4: Fluency Client

Subjective: Doug was in a good mood today. He was excited about the upcoming spring break.

Objective:

STO 1: The client will utilize smooth controlled speech during a structured reading task (words, phrases, sentences) with 80% accuracy.

Data: 9/10 = 90%(words)
6/10 = 60% (phrases)
6/10 = 60% (sentences)

STO 2: The client will reduce disfluencies to less than 20% during a 3-minute conversation with a familiar person in the therapy room.

Data: 19% (15/80) in 2 minutes of conversation

STO 3: The client will reduce disfluencies to less than 20% when speaking to an unfamiliar person in the therapy room.

Data: 26% (100/386) in 10 minutes of conversation

Assessment: Doug's reading at the phrase and sentence level was not as fluent as usual. He stated that he did not focus on being "as relaxed as he should have." He still felt that "overall, it was pretty good." He had difficulty when speaking with Alex, an unfamiliar person, and admitted that his blocks were longer and more frequent because he wasn't using his techniques. He appears to be motivated by tracking his progress on a weekly graph.

Plan: Videotape the next session to allow for more feedback and continue to talk to him about his self-monitoring skills. Choose stimuli for reading that does not contain problematic words in order to increase success. Continue to bring in an unfamiliar person to engage Doug in conversation.

These are just a few examples of what a SOAP note looks like. As mentioned previously, the SOAP format is used in many different settings and will vary in length, detail, and content, depending on the setting. Additional examples of SOAP notes are included in Appendix S.

MEDICAL SETTINGS

Many of the medical professionals we interviewed informed us that it is often the case that students are timid or hesitant when writing information in a patient's chart. They seem to be afraid of writing the wrong information, writing too much information, or not writing enough information. It is our goal to help you know what to write, and how to write it, so this won't happen to you.

As mentioned previously, SOAP notes are standard documentation for many different medical professionals. In a hospital, nursing home, or rehab hospital, doctors, nurses, and rehab staff (therapists) may all use SOAP notes to communicate regarding a patient's care. Therefore, many of the SOAP notes found in a patient's chart may look similar. What will distinguish a speech-language SOAP note from a medical SOAP note will be the goals that are written in the Objective section. What will distinguish a speech-language SOAP note in a medical facility from a speech-language SOAP note anywhere else is the medical terminology that will be contained therein. We feel it's worth explaining a few terms, abbreviations, and symbols that you may encounter in a medical setting. Appendix K lists commonly used symbols and abbreviations and their meaning. Due to the limited amount of space, as well as the number of professionals who add information to a patient's medical chart, you can appreciate the need for the SLP in a medical setting to use abbreviations and symbols as often as possible.

Because patients requiring SLP services at a medical facility have likely recently experienced one or more major medical events, have multiple diagnoses, or multiple comoribidities, you will be using abbreviations outside of those related to communication skills. When working in a medical facility, you are strongly warned to only use approved abbreviations so all those reading the chart will understand precisely what you are communicating. For example, if you are recommending that a patient be "NPO" due to severe dysphagia, you want to be sure to use the appropriate abbreviation so as not to misconstrue this information, and endanger your patient. In addition to using abbreviations in your paperwork, you will need to identify abbreviations when reading about your patient in the chart. Understanding abbreviations is vital when making evaluation and treatment decisions about your patient. Learning abbreviations for medical conditions such as COPD (chronic obstructive pulmonary disease) and GERD (gastroesophageal reflux disease) is important as this might indicate a need for a swallowing evaluation. When you encounter an abbreviation with which you are not familiar, do not risk of guessing but take the time to look up the term. There is typically a dictionary of medical abbreviations and terms at the nurses' station.

Depending on the facility, terminology used in documentation may vary based on the type of system used to measure a patient's progress. As we mentioned in Chapter 5, it is common to see *functional independence measures* or FIM scores. This system, as the name implies, evaluates patients based on their level of independence.

We have found that most facilities use this system or one that is similar. Some facilities may only use the numbers from the FIM scale or similar abbreviations. For instance, they may write, "Pt. will improve comprehension from level 4 to level 5," or they may use MOD or MIN rather than MIN-A (minimum assistance) or MOD-I (modified independent). In general, the criteria are the same even if the abbreviations vary. Let's take a look at what a SLP note might actually look like in a rehabilitation setting. The following SOAP note is for a patient who

is working on memory, intelligibility, and problem-solving using a functional independence rating.

Subjective: Pt. seen for 2 units of speech tx today; pt. alert & cooperative with no complaint of pain.

Objective: Pt. completed OMEs c̄ SPV, to ↑ labial and lingual ROM. Pt. able to recall 2/3 speech strategies and completed speech intelligibility tasks at imitative sentence level c̄ MIN-A. Pt required mod cues to provide solutions for problems related to ADLs.

Assessment: Independence with OMEs ↑ today, less cueing needed for intelligibility tasks, and increased cueing needed for problem-solving tasks as situations were more complex.

Plan: Continue POC.

Due to daily caseload numbers, lack of space in the medical chart, and the number of people who have to read the information, most speech pathology notes in a medical setting are brief and use similar terminology. This is true for other therapists as well as nurses, doctors, and other professional staff, making it even more important that the SLP in a medical setting become familiar with all types of terminology. It is vital that you only use approved abbreviations, as using an abbreviation that someone else is unfamiliar with may result in confusion and a failure to communicate.

Keep in mind that as a student clinician, when you sign any documentation, a licensed SLP will be required to sign as well. Therefore, even if you are unsure about what to write, your supervisor will review and sign off on your note. When learning how to best document your patient's goals and progress, you should remember the common adage, "If it is not written in the patient's chart, it didn't happen." While your notes and reports will not be as lengthy as in the university clinic, it is still vital to document certain aspects of evaluation and treatment.

PUBLIC SCHOOL SETTINGS

Due to the federally mandated use of the Individualized Education Program (IEP), the SOAP note is not a staple of reporting in the public schools. Most SLPs who work in the public schools devise their own system to track data and simply report final data in the section of the IEP form that is designated specifically for reporting progress. Methods of data collection may vary greatly among school systems, schools within the same system, or individual therapists. As a practicum student in the public schools, you will be expected to follow the system that your particular school has in place. This may mean that you will use specific data collection forms or that you design your own form; each school will be different.

Even though forms and procedures may differ across school systems, what remains the same is how each child's progress is reported on the actual IEP form. This is federally mandated, and therefore not open to interpretation.

We have provided a sample Annual Goal Progress Report form that is used in our local school system (Appendix N). You will notice that there are six reporting periods, as well as a legend in the middle of the page that is used to evaluate the student's progress toward the annual goals. This information is of paramount importance in determining changes to be made to the IEP when it is updated each year and must be documented on the IEP during the designated reporting period. This designated "progress reporting" period may not be the same across school systems. In the State of Alabama, progress must be documented on the student's IEP every 9 weeks; however, your particular school's requirements may be different.

Progress reporting is a necessary component of the delivery of SLP services. Becoming efficient at reporting progress or lack thereof, regardless of the setting in which you eventually practice, is a crucial skill to develop as a student clinician and one that will only enhance your clinical skills throughout your professional career.

7 Long-Term Progress Reports

Our goal as speech-language pathologists is to help our clients attain (to the greatest extent possible) normal function of their speech, language, or swallowing abilities. In order to accomplish this task, we must gather reliable data that measure and validate this change over time. As we have discussed in previous chapters, these data are what determines if we have achieved our goals through the delivery of speech-language pathology services, as well as our ability to receive payment or reimbursement (from a third-party payer) for those services. Now that we have shown you how to write goals, objectives, daily notes, and short-term progress reports, we would be remiss if we did not discuss how to report progress for patients who are in therapy for an extended period of time. Long-term progress reports summarize information that has most likely been documented in previous documentation such as daily notes and/or short-term progress notes. This chapter provides setting-specific information on long-term progress reports as well as information about discharge summaries, when they are needed, and what they look like.

UNIVERSITY CLINIC

Due to the nature of how treatment takes place in a university clinic, namely, that clients receive treatment for the duration of a quarter or semester, the long-term progress report generally serves as a summary for the therapy term. In addition to the daily SOAP or weekly progress notes, most training programs require students to prepare a final report that includes data for all of the client's goals for the entire term. This document may be referred to as a final treatment report or progress report, depending on the university program and the terminology it chooses to use. Most clients who attend a university clinic for speech-language services expect these reports, as do other allied professionals who collaborate with clinicians in university clinics.

For example, if a child is receiving services in the public school as well as at the university clinic, a copy of the long-term progress report is usually sent to the school SLP in order to ensure that both parties are addressing the same needs for the child. Also, if a client has been referred to the university clinic by another professional (psychologist, physician, occupational therapist, etc.), it is standard practice to send that individual a copy of the client's progress report with a note thanking him for the referral. If a client is being seen by a number of different professionals, this sharing of information can be vital in the overall treatment of the client.

The long-term progress report is important for several reasons, which we explain below. This may include, but is not limited to:

1. Short-term and long-term progress reporting is required by ASHA and third-party payers.

   All university programs must abide by certain ASHA guidelines in order to maintain their accreditation. These guidelines stipulate that a variety of documentation must be in place on a consistent basis. Students must keep an accurate record of their clinical hours, and there must be a system in place to keep up with each client's progress. Most clinics have a confidential file system, in which each client has a personal and confidential file that is kept in a secure location.

At the end of each term, treatment reports or long-term progress reports must be placed in the client's file for safekeeping. ASHA requires this confidential filing system, as does the federal government, due to enactment of the Health Information Portability and Accountability Act (HIPAA). As far as billing is concerned, if a clinic bills Medicaid, Medicare, or private insurance, accurate records ensure that these entities are being billed for valid service delivery. Any discrepancies in paperwork can result in denial of payment for services and this reflects poorly on the program, the clinic, and the university.

2. Clients may remain in therapy for several semesters, or even years and a record should be kept of past performance.

It is not uncommon for many patients (especially adults) in a university clinic to end up there due to an insurance company being unwilling to continue paying for services through a hospital or private practitioner. As we discussed in an earlier chapter, third-party payers usually stipulate the exact number of sessions they will cover relating to any type of rehabilitation therapy. Once the patient has completed the designated number of sessions, he must find services elsewhere or pay out-of-pocket expenses. And, due to the fact that university clinics are training facilities, many operate on a sliding fee scale, based on a client's income. It is also necessary that students have clients for whom they can provide services in order for the clinical training program to thrive. Therefore, some clients will remain in therapy for an extended period of time due to the reduced or waived fees and willingness of the clinical staff at the university clinic to work with them.

3. Clients often have a new student clinician each semester, and historical data are important when planning treatment each term.

Most university training programs have the goal of providing student clinicians with the most diverse clinical experience possible, allowing them to work with both children and adults in a variety of disorder areas. This is usually accomplished through practicum experience in the university clinic as well as off-campus sites. It is for this reason that clients are often seen in the university clinic that have been discharged from other private practitioners, hospitals, or rehabilitation facilities, due to insurance reasons or lack of progress. Generally, clients in the university clinic will have a new student clinician each semester in order for students to receive training in all disorder areas. This is especially true for a client with a less common disorder. In order for the new clinician to best prepare to treat the client, a thorough review of previous long-term reports is necessary. This sheds light on what progress has been made or lack thereof, and the use of certain therapy approaches, cues, reinforcement, and procedures. Much time can be saved when attempting to craft the most efficient and effective treatment plan by reviewing long-term reports.

4. The client and/or parent or caregiver is provided with a record of progress.

Just as you expect a report from a physician or specialist when you have any type of testing or treatment done, your clients expect the same information regarding the speech therapy services you have provided. Not only are clients/parents given progress reports in order to summarize data for themselves or their child's therapy sessions, in the case of older children and adults, but the progress report may serve as a tool to motivate the clients to continue with therapy until maximum potential is achieved.

It is important to add here that many times, the long-term progress report will also serve as a discharge summary. If a client is being discharged from therapy, this is usually mentioned in the "Recommendations" section of the report. For example, "Based on Mr. Smith meeting criteria over the past 3 sessions, it is recommended that he be discharged from speech therapy at this time." More than likely, your clinic will have protocols in place for how and when to write progress/treatment reports, and your clinical supervisors will assist you in this process. However, we provide an example of a university clinic long-term treatment report in Appendix O.

MEDICAL SETTINGS

Due to the nature of treatment across various medical settings, we address each one separately in this section.

Rehabilitation Hospital

As we mentioned in Chapter 4, patients are typically admitted to a rehabilitation hospital for a predetermined amount of time. This depends on the patient's level of functioning, often referred to as *burden of care*, as well as their insurance coverage. Persons aged 65 or older are eligible for Medicare, whereas patients under the age of 65 must rely on private insurance or pay expenses out of pocket. The average stay for Medicare patients is 14 days, although patients who have private insurance may stay longer, depending on how much time their insurance company will allow. At the culmination of their stay in the rehabilitation facility, one of three things will happen. They are (a) discharged home or to a caregiver's home, (b) transferred to the hospital, or (c) admitted to a long-term care facility.

As was evident in the chapter on writing long-term and short-term goals, some facilities do not even bother to write long-term goals, although others have a long-term goal, but the outcomes reflect what one could reasonably expect to accomplish during a 2-week period. For example, a client in a university clinic may have a long-term goal of returning to work on a part-time basis following a stroke or TBI, whereas this same individual may have a long-term goal of following multistep directions with minimal assistance while in the rehabilitation facility. You may want to refer back to Chapter 5 for examples of long-term goals for each type of medical facility. The progress report for these patients will reflect not only the goals that were targeted, but also the amount of time the patient spends working on these goals.

A long-term progress report may also serve as the discharge report for a patient who has only spent 14 days in a rehabilitation facility. The discharge summary may be the same form that was used for reporting the patient's progress and will also use functional independence measures (FIM) scores to indicate the patient's status at discharge. At times, the SLP may actually discharge a patient from speech and language therapy before he is discharged from a facility. Whenever the client is discharged from SLP services, whether during their stay or at the conclusion, you will generally write a *discharge note or summary* on a specific form. Along with discharge instructions, you may fill out a Patient Education section that indicates what information you have provided to the patient regarding any necessary home care or home program.

Hospital

Similar to the rehabilitation setting, a patient's stay in a hospital may be very limited. Very often, patients are seen in acute care for just a few days until they are stable enough to be moved to the rehabilitation wing of the hospital, another rehabilitation facility, or discharged home. As a general rule, patients do not have long-term goals in acute care; it is the goal of the medical professionals working with patients in acute care to get them medically stable so that they can participate in and benefit from any therapies they may need once they recover. The SLP who sees a critically ill patient in acute care may be there only to do a bedside swallowing evaluation to determine if the patient is safe to eat a normal diet, needs diet modifications, or needs alternative means of nutrition.

Once the patient is stable, the physician will write an order for the SLP evaluation. Once this evaluation has been completed and the patient's needs are determined, the SLP will then write appropriate goals for the patient and begin treatment. You may refer back to Chapter 5 for examples of short-term and long-term goals in a hospital setting.

Long-Term Care Facility/Nursing Home

Unless they have been temporarily transferred to the nursing home until they recover enough function to return home, most patients who are in long-term care may remain there for the duration of their life. Even though these patients may remain in the long-term care facility a very long time, they will only qualify for speech-language therapy for a specific amount of time. Therefore, long-term progress reports for these patients are very similar to those of the acute care or rehabilitation hospital. The SLP often uses appropriate goals from a *goal bank* and then selects short-term objectives as a way to achieve the long-term goal. Once again, goals must be functional in order for the facility to be reimbursed by Medicare or other third-party payers — if the patient is not making progress, the case cannot be made that he should continue receiving services. The long-term goal will most likely be written so that it may be achieved in the time frame that has been stipulated by payment for services. Please refer to Appendix Q for an example of a progress note used in a long-term care facility.

SCHOOL SETTINGS

If you find yourself assigned to a practicum in the public schools, you will become very familiar with the *Individualized Education Program* (IEP). With the information provided in Chapter 5, along with the experience you gain first hand, you will begin to develop an understanding of how the IEP functions.

The IEP has a built-in system for tracking progress. Recall from Chapter 5 that benchmarks are developed for each long-term goal that stipulate a time frame for each goal to be achieved. Personnel responsible for implementing the IEP must then report the student's progress to the parent or guardian of the child who is receiving services on a regular basis. Due to the nature of this periodic reporting system, there is no long-term progress report for children who are being served through the public schools — progress is reported at various intervals throughout the school year, such as every 6 or 9 weeks, and then the parent(s), teachers, special education teachers, and other professionals meet once a year to discuss how the child has progressed based on the benchmarks set forth from the previous year's meeting. In this way, each person who is responsible for implementing the IEP will understand the ultimate academic goal for this child.

It is probably fairly clear to you now that reporting progress is a mainstay in the field of SLP. Without reports of how our clients are performing, we have no way to determine if we should stay the course, modify treatment, or discharge someone from therapy altogether. The long-term progress report tells us if the long-term goal (the ultimate outcome we want for our clients) is being achieved, and if not, how we should proceed in the future.

8 Professional Correspondence

Although we have discussed many forms of written communication that you will be expected to master during your clinical training, one that we have not addressed is professional correspondence. In the course of a normal work week the speech-language pathologist will generate a variety of different types of correspondence in addition to the report writing we have discussed in previous chapters. Whether you are writing referral letters, transmittal letters, thank-you letters, e-mails, or memoranda, the ability to communicate effectively will speak volumes about your knowledge, clinical competence, organization, and professionalism. In short, you will establish credibility with professional and well-written communication. Professionalism is not just reserved for our verbal interactions and clinical reports; it shows up in our written correspondence as well.

How does your written communication project an image of you? Imagine if you will that you are a parent whose child is receiving speech-language therapy at the university clinic. You receive a letter from the student who has been working with your child, and in the first paragraph, there are two typographical errors and a run-on sentence. What is your impression going to be? Would you think that this student is professional or unorganized? Would you wonder if this graduate student's lack of attention to detail might carry over to her preparation for your child's therapy? We feel the latter would be true. The way we communicate, whether verbally or in writing, truly says a lot about us as professionals.

During your time in school, you will be required to demonstrate two types of writing: academic and clinical. Academic writing includes research papers, term papers, journal reviews, or even answers to comprehensive test questions. Clinical writing encompasses all of the reports and documents we have covered thus far in this text, in addition to the type of correspondence we address in this chapter—e-mails, referral letters, and the like. Although you are expected to come into the university with some basic writing skills that enable you to complete these academic writing tasks, we understand that clinical writing is a unique genre of communication. Most students will not come into a training program with knowledge of professional clinical writing. This is a skill you will acquire right along with the clinical competencies you develop toward becoming a certified SLP.

THE BASICS

Professional writing is a challenging yet important and necessary part of your training. Lack of student preparedness in training programs is nothing new, however; the authors have learned through interviews with practicum supervisors and in professional seminars that students' writing skills are frequently an area of weakness. In other words, this is a problem all students and training programs have to face.

University training programs will address this issue in various ways, and it is our hope that you will have the support you need to become proficient in your professional writing abilities. Unfortunately, there typically is no formal course in clinical writing at most universities, and many students have not received adequate writing practice in general. Although students may have the opportunity to write term papers, essays, or journal reviews, they have not had any practice with clinical writing until they are thrust into it once they begin clinical practicum. Even then, they are at the mercy of varied supervisors who have different ideas about the level of writing skill they should possess. This is made even more complicated because supervisors may differ in their own styles of clinical writing.

It is interesting to note that one university in Florida started a pilot course in clinical writing skills in order to address the lack of knowledge and experience of its students in speech-language pathology. It was also instructive that one of the recommendations following implementation of this pilot course was the development of a "sample report book" that students could follow. According to Middleton et al. (1992), "Providing students with sample reports and training exercises allows more training in the recognition of good writing." So, even though writing prowess improves with practice and experience, there is obviously a need for guidelines and examples of what a professionally written document should look like. This same concept applies to professional correspondence such as letters and memoranda.

Organization

All well-written documents must be organized in such a way that makes them easy to follow. How many times have you read and reread something, only to find that you still cannot discern the meaning the writer is attempting to convey? When it comes to drafting a professional document, organization includes everything from sentence structure to word usage to placement of information within the document. Most resources you find that address organizational aspects of professional writing will include a list of "must-haves" for a professional document (Strunk & White, 2000). Many guidelines used in writing business reports include some key components that relate to the business letters, thank-you letters, transmittal letters, and referral letters discussed in this chapter. In the next section, we provide examples of some of these documents; however, we would like to introduce the following information to you at this time, as we feel it is relevant to organization and it applies to various types of correspondence.

- The letter should be written on letterhead stationery if it is from a clinical facility.

- Every piece of professional correspondence should be dated at the top.

- There should be an inside address that includes basic information such as the name, address, and affiliation of the intended recipient of the letter.

- The letter should include a professional and respectful greeting or salutation (e.g., Dear Mrs. Johnson).

- The first paragraph of the letter typically provides some background information about the sender so that the recipient of the letter knows something about the person generating the correspondence.

- The body of the letter or memo should contain the reason the document is being written and whom it is written about. It should be broken up into logical paragraphs or subheadings, if necessary.

- There should be a summary or conclusion paragraph reiterating the purpose of the letter and thanking the recipient for her consideration in reading the document.

- Prior to the signature line there should be what is known as a *complimentary closing* (e.g., "Sincerely, Respectfully").

- The signature line should include the typed name of the sender, her degrees, and position. In the case of students you can refer to yourself as "student clinician," "graduate clinician," or the like.

Let us now take a look at how this organizational structure applies to the various types of communication we have mentioned. In general, there are four types of letters that you may be required to write during your clinical training: referral letters, thank-you letters, transmittal (cover) letters, and business letters. These are explained further below:

- **Referral Letter:** This will usually accompany a diagnostic or treatment report for a client you are referring to another professional for services not within the scope of practice of the SLP. For example, we routinely refer clients to physicians, psychologists, occupational therapists, physical therapists, special educators, social workers, regular educators, and audiologists, among others. This letter describes the reason for the referral and introduces the client to the professional to whom we are referring the case. Without some explanation, the professional would be at a loss to understand the purpose of the referral.

▧ **Thank-You Letter:** This will usually be sent as a follow-up when a client has been referred to you from another professional. Expressing your appreciation for the referral will hopefully serve to maintain a positive professional relationship and may result in more referrals in the future. Thank-you letters are also appropriate when a company sends you complementary materials or someone donates toys/materials to your clinic. Such letters are also used when other professionals donate their time and expertise to consult with you on a case. It is a good policy to thank people for any contributions of time, materials, or finances.

▧ **Transmittal or Cover Letter:** This usually accompanies a diagnostic or treatment report that is being sent to a professional, client, parent, or caregiver. It is not professional to simply mail a report to someone without a letter of explanation accompanying the document. Such cover letters explain why the report is being sent.

▧ **Business Letter:** This is used when writing to a company or organization in order to request a service or materials. We also use business letters to correspond with insurance companies and businesses that provide administrative support to clinics such as office supplies, copying machines, and clerical personnel. Business letters might also be used to make other professionals aware of existing clinical programs offered by your facility or announce the establishment of new services by the clinic.

All four of the letters mentioned above require organization, a specific format, and professional communication. The letters sent by the SLP not only represent the individual practitioner, but the facility for which she or he works, so they must be professionally done.

An example of each type of letter is provided below.

Sample Referral Letter

August 2, 2012

Jennifer Smith, OT
Main Street Rehabilitation
Montgomery, AL

Dear Ms. Smith:

I am writing this letter in regard to Sam Jones, a 3-year-old male, who was seen at this clinic for a speech and language evaluation on July 23, 2012. Sam was referred to us by his pediatrician due to a speech and language delay. During the case history interview, Janice Jones, Sam's mother, also described several other behaviors that are causing her quite a bit of concern.

Based on results of our assessment, Sam does exhibit a language delay; however, he is also demonstrating self-stimulating behaviors such as spinning and diverted eye gaze. Mrs. Jones reports that Sam is also a very "picky" eater, and that he "does not like things touching him." Based on results of our evaluation, as well as his mother's concerns, we feel that a comprehensive occupational therapy evaluation is warranted.

I appreciate your assessment of this very interesting child and am enclosing a copy of our diagnostic report for your review. I look forward to receiving your input on this case.

Sincerely,

Embry Burrus, MCD, CCC/SLP
Associate Clinical Professor

Enclosure

Sample Thank-You Letter

August 2, 2012

Daniel Rice, M.D.
Regional Medical Clinic
123 Main St.
Auburn, AL 36830

Dear Dr. Rice:

Thank you for referring James Goodwin to our clinic for a speech and language evaluation. We completed our evaluation of James on July 25, 2012, and have recommended that he receive speech therapy here at our clinic for the upcoming semester.

Our findings indicate that James continues to exhibit language and pragmatic difficulties as a result of the TBI he sustained approximately one year ago. Your assessment of his social language skills was excellent, and we appreciate your insight into this matter. Once we have James's authorization, we will be happy to send you a progress report at the end of the semester. Should you have any questions, or need further information, please contact us at your convenience.

Once again, thank you for your referral.

Sincerely,

Heather Daniels, B.S.
Student Clinician

Sample Transmittal Letter

August 7, 2012

Jennifer Smith, OT
Main Street Rehabilitation
Montgomery, AL

Dear Ms. Smith:

Enclosed please find the diagnostic report for Sam Smith, a 3-year-old male, who was evaluated at this clinic on July 30, 2012. Per our phone conversation, Sam has been referred to your clinic for occupational therapy due to sensory integration disorder and decreased fine motor skills.

Should you need any further information, please contact us at (123) 456-7890. I look forward to hearing from you and collaborating with you in the treatment of this child.

Sincerely,

Amy Sellers, B.S.
Student Clinician

Enclosure

Sample Business Letter

August 7, 2012

Daniel Means, President
Therapy Works, Inc.
123 Main St.
Birmingham, AL

Dear Mr. Means:

My name is Ann Smith, and I am a graduate student in speech-language pathology at Ourtown University. I am very interested in learning more about the therapy materials that you offer for children who have feeding and swallowing disorders. I am about to begin my externship at a pediatric clinic and expect to see a number of children who have been diagnosed with these disorders.

I read in your catalog that a representative from your company will come to our university and demonstrate the products and that you offer a discount if we make a purchase following the demonstration. I would appreciate any assistance you could provide in arranging this for our students.

Thank you for your time and attention to this matter. I may be reached at (123) 456-9900, or via e-mail at a.smith@ourtown.edu. I look forward to hearing from you very soon.

Sincerely,

Ann Smith, B.S.
Student in SLP
Ourtown University

Another form of written correspondence you may use is the memorandum, or "memo." The memo is standard business correspondence, and, before the advent of electronic mail, was used more often by people communicating in work settings than any other type of written correspondence. The memo is still widely used today; so often, in fact, that you will hear references made to it throughout virtually every communication medium—television, radio, and water cooler conversations when people say, "Didn't you get the memo?"

The memorandum was designed to transmit important information in a brief, concise format.

According to the *Merriam-Webster Dictionary*, the definition of memorandum is: "a usually brief communication written for interoffice circulation; a communication that contains directive, advisory or informative matter." Thus, memoranda typically are not sent outside of the office in which you are working to other facilities. The memos you will be required to write will generally serve one of three purposes: (a) transmitting information, (b) requesting information, or (c) requesting or enabling action. We provide a couple of examples in the boxes.

Requesting or Enabling Action

MEMORANDUM

To: Beverly Jones, Office Manager
Fr: Ashley Smith, Graduate Student, SLP
Re: Confidential file
Date: 8-4-12

I am writing to inform you that I am in receipt of paperwork from the graduate school that needs to be added to my personal and confidential file. I understand that you only receive information from students at specific times. Please let me know when would be a good time for me to get this information to you. Thank you for your assistance in this matter.

Transmitting Information

MEMORANDUM

To: Dr. Ron Good, Department Chair
Fr: Ashley Smith, Graduate Student, SLP
Re: Comprehensive Exams
Date: 9-12-12

I am writing in regard to the oral comprehensive exam that I missed due to a death in my family. At your convenience, I would like to meet with you in order to discuss a time to reschedule this exam. Thank you for your understanding and assistance in this matter.

What you are most likely thinking at this point is that you would probably send an e-mail in each one of these cases; and, most likely, you would be right. As a matter of fact, electronic mail has, in many cases, taken the place of the interoffice memoran-

dum. On many campuses, e-mail is considered an "official" communication between faculty, staff, and students. Therefore, students have the responsibility of checking their e-mail daily for communications from faculty members or the university administration. It is no excuse to say that you did not read your e-mail if an assignment is given to the class via this form of communication. Often, e-mail is exchanged between facilities for the purpose of scheduling appointments or other tasks associated with clients. In making this point, we would like to add that your e-mails, when used in the same way as the previous memo examples, should be just as well written and organized. We emphasize that you resist the temptation to use "text message" speech, abbreviations, and slang. This is not professional and will communicate to whoever receives your message a lack of professionalism. Do not make the mistake of communicating something about yourself that you do not intend. It is also wise to remember that any information transmitted electronically is susceptible to eavesdropping by hackers and others, especially if you are communicating over an unsecure connection and using nonencrypted e-mail. As we mentioned in an earlier chapter, you could be violating a client's confidentiality by sending sensitive clinical information by e-mail if it is intercepted by an unintended recipient. People can also easily access another person's computer and read e-mail that is stored on that machine or simply look over a shoulder and read the screen. The bottom line is that you must be very careful transmitting client information via e-mail. This also applies to sending clinical reports as e-mail attachments.

In this next section, we would like to mention a few aspects of writing to keep in mind when you are putting together your written communication.

Format

Using an outline each time you write will ensure the correct structure or format of your document, and generally, structure is one thing that does not change, regardless of who you are writing to or about. If you think back to when you learned to write a letter in grade school, you will recall that you were given an outline that you could use each time you sat down to write: the date in the top left or right corner, followed by the person's name and address to whom you were writing, the salutation, the body of the letter, and then, at the bottom of the page, the name of the sender. This was standard "letter writing" format, and you probably committed it to memory fairly easily. Our intention is to make the process of professional writing just as easy to learn, so that once you have mastered it, you will take that skill with you into the work setting you choose.

Tone and Language

The feeling you get when reading a document is mostly related to the tone in which the writer is communicating. Tone is sometimes referred to as the "voice" or "attitude" of a piece of writing. Voice, however, may also refer to the tense you are writing in, such as passive or active. Generally, professional documents are written in the passive voice. For example, "Michael was observed to use several multiword utterances," as opposed to "Michael said four three-word sentences."

In an earlier chapter we mentioned *professional tone* as applied to writing reports. This applies to writing professional correspondence as well. If you read a letter, e-mail, or memorandum that appears to be immature, nonchalant, or informal, you may wonder about the professionalism of the writer. So the words you choose to use, as well as the structure of your document, will convey a specific tone, and you always want that tone to be professional. For example, you might say, "Michael has difficulty staying on task, which may have a negative effect on his success in therapy," as opposed to "Michael won't pay attention and wiggles in his chair." The tone of each of these sentences is very different, not only because of the voice, but also because of the words that are used; "has difficulty staying on task" sounds professional, whereas "wiggles in his chair" does not. It may be helpful to refer to the term generator we have provided to find appropriate professional terminology. As we alluded to earlier, it is important to have a good working knowledge of professional terminology, as you will use it frequently when writing clinical documents. It is also important, however, that

information is communicated in a clear, concise manner (French & Sim, 1993). In addition, you want your communication to be appropriate for the person who will be receiving it. A letter that is being sent to a parent will not always read the same as information sent to a physician or other health care professional. Your reader should not need a dictionary, medical or otherwise, or an advanced degree to understand your letter. It has been our experience that students get so caught up in using the professional jargon they have learned that they want to "show it off." Professional terminology is not written for the purpose of impressing others with your knowledge. When communicating with other professionals, it can be a way to write detailed information in an abbreviated manner, but when communicating with parents or caregivers, it is a way to describe the results of your treatment or assessment in a way that is easy to understand—the goal is clear communication of sometimes complicated ideas. In his book *On Writing Well*, William K. Zinsser makes this point when he writes (Zinsser, 2006, p. 8):

Perhaps the sentence is so excessively cluttered, that the reader, hacking through the verbiage, simply doesn't know what it means. Perhaps a sentence is so shoddily constructed that the reader does not know how to read it, or perhaps Sentence B is not a logical sequence to Sentence A.

Finally, you should always pay attention to the grammar and organization of professional letters and to spelling, as well. Fortunately, most word processing programs have grammar and spell-checking tools that will alert you to your linguistic missteps, but remember that these programs are not infallible as demonstrated by the anonymous poem in the box below.

Spell Checker Blues

Eye halve a spelling chequer
It came with my pea sea
It plainly marques four my revue
Miss steaks eye kin knot sea.

Eye strike a key and type a word
And weight four it two say

Weather eye am wrong oar write
It shows me strait a weigh.

As soon as a mist ache is maid
It nose bee fore two long
And eye can put the error rite
Its rarely ever wrong.

Eye have run this poem threw it
I am shore your pleased two no
Its letter perfect in it's weigh
My chequer tolled me sew.

Anon.

The purpose of the present chapter has been to bring to a conscious level the notion that *any* written communication generated by the SLP puts forth an image of professionalism. The reports, letters, memoranda, and e-mails that you produce reflect not only on you as a professional, but on the facility you represent. They must be organized in the correct format, written in professional language, and free of grammatical and spelling errors. Do not hesitate to take the opportunity to carefully review the documents you generate, because once you hit the "Enter" button or drop that envelope in the mailbox, it is far too late for revisions.

SECTION III

Professional Verbal Communication

9 Interacting with Clients and Families

In the previous section of this text we discussed professional written communication in the form of diagnostic reports, treatment plans, and various forms of progress reports. Your written communications have a profound effect on how you are perceived by others and they also serve to guide your clinical work. As a student in speech-language pathology, you will be using professional written communication across various practicum settings and we hope that the general guidelines we have provided in prior chapters will serve you well. A book about professional communication, however, should discuss more than just the writing of reports. Communication takes place through several modalities and writing is only one of them. You will find that in every practicum setting, you will participate in verbal interactions with clients, family members, other professionals, and clinical supervisors. In most cases, these verbal interactions between people have an even greater impact on your clients, other professionals, and supervisors than your written reports. Verbal interactions are pivotal in the way you are perceived by others and central to how clients, families, professionals, and supervisors form an opinion about your professionalism. Do not underestimate the importance of each verbal interaction you have with others because these exchanges have a significant impact in two critical areas. First, as stated above, verbal interactions are the primary determinant of another person's perception of you as a professional. Second, we use verbal interactions to gain information, counsel clients, provide information, and train others to participate in the treatment process. Although we could do all of these things in written communication, there would be no opportunity for exchange of information between the clinician and others. Clients and other professionals have questions that must be answered by the clinician. In many cases, it is important to convince clients and professionals to participate in the treatment program and motivate them to perform for greater progress in therapy. Perhaps more significantly, verbal communication adds the all-important human element to clinical practice. Face-to-face verbal interactions can often be the critical variable in success or failure of a treatment effort.

Your program may or may not have a course dedicated to the area of counseling or devote much time to verbal communication. Regardless, it is an area in which you will need to refine your skills to best serve your clients. This chapter is designed to be an introduction to the foundations of effective and professional verbal communication and to review the varied aspects of interaction between you and those that you serve. ASHA (2012) calls us to be responsible for this in its scope of practice document, which states that SLPs are responsible for "educating and counseling individuals, families, coworkers, educators, and other persons in the community regarding acceptance, adaptation, and decision making about communication and swallowing." Please note that when we refer to the "client" in this chapter, we are being inclusive of any caregivers you may be speaking with as well, including parents, grandparents, or spouses of the clients.

SELECTED CRITICAL ELEMENTS OF PROFESSIONAL VERBAL COMMUNICATION

From examining the table of contents you know that we present four separate chapters on professional verbal communication. This chapter focuses on communication with clients. The next three chapters address communication issues related to other professionals, individuals from diverse backgrounds, and clinical supervisors. There are, however, some critical elements that should be infused in professional verbal communication across all of these groups. Thus, while we discuss these variables here, you should remember that they should be part of all professional verbal communication. There are many other characteristics that have been suggested over the years that contribute to effective interviewing and counseling. For example, Shipley (1997) lists the following: sensitivity, respect, empathy, objectivity, listening skills, motivation, and rapport. Many of these are subsumed under the five elements we discuss below. We have chosen only five variables because they are probably among the most impor-

tant for beginning clinicians, and they relate to professional communication. Figure 9–1 illustrates five factors that should be present in all professional interactions and we briefly discuss each of them in the following sections.

Show Respect

This component is something that should be part of any communication, whether professional or casual, but it is especially important for clinicians (Shipley, 1997). We want our clients, other professionals, and clinical supervisors to feel as if they are treated with respect for their infinite dignity and worth as human beings. Clients and families come to us for services to ameliorate a communication disorder that is hav-

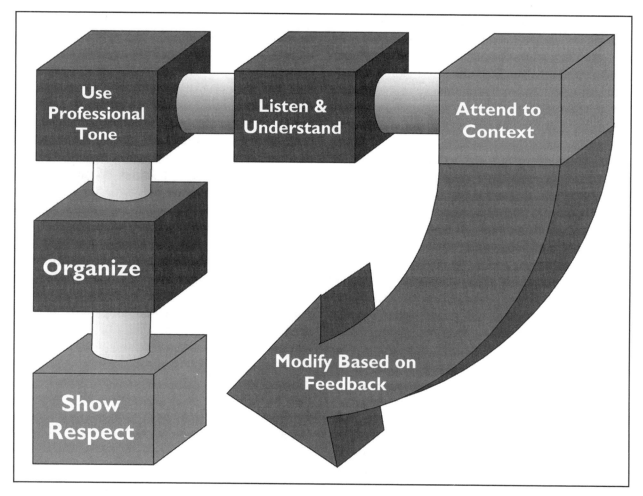

Figure 9–1. Selected critical elements of professional verbal communication.

ing a negative impact on their lives. They may feel embarrassed and at a disadvantage when they have to come to a professional for help. We ask them for personal information about their problems, which again makes them feel vulnerable. These clients need to believe that the professional will treat them and the information they provide with dignity and respect. So how do we behave when we treat clients respectfully? First, it is common that at the beginning of the clinical relationship we refer to clients with a respectful term of address such as "Mr. Jones" or "Mrs. Smith." This form of address connotes a professional relationship and communicates respect for the client/family member. Obviously, after working with a family for a period of time you become more familiar and the person may say, "Please, call me Michelle." It is then appropriate to refer to the client/ family member as he or she wishes, but we believe that it should be their call. Imagine yourself in a hospital after having a stroke. You have been deprived of all dignity and are in a vulnerable position. Then a stranger comes into your room and says, "How ya doin', Charlie?" This kind of familiarity from someone you have never met is not a respectful form of address. It is much more professional to say something like, "Hello, Mr. Smith, I'm Suzanne Jones, a speech therapist. I understand you've had a stroke and are having some trouble talking." Just by using a term such as "Mr. Smith," you have communicated respect for the patient. When dealing with other professionals it is always good to begin by using their title (e.g., Dr. Smith) or calling them "Mr.," "Mrs.," or "Ms." You will find yourself working with psychologists, physicians, teachers, physical therapists, occupational therapists, and many other professionals who are consulting on your client. When you are at a staffing or introducing other professionals to family members, referring to them more formally is a sign of respect. As everyone gets to know each other, you will know when to refer to other professionals less formally. Regarding verbal communication with supervisors, it goes without saying that you want to strike a respectful posture with someone who is evaluating your practicum performance.

Respect for a person is also communicated nonverbally and by the physical environment in which you communicate. Your nonverbal behavior should suggest that you are genuinely interested in his concerns and take the interaction very seriously. You should conduct professional communications in a comfortable, professional environment that protects client confidentiality and provides an opportunity for the person to express himself without distractions. Making a person comfortable in a professional environment shows that you respect him as an individual and care about his concerns.

Organize

You will recall from Chapter 8 that we suggested that one of the most important parts of writing diagnostic reports is organization. Having an organization to the information you provide makes the report follow a logical sequence and increases its intelligibility to the reader. It is exactly the same with professional verbal communication. No one wants to listen to a person who just rambles on in an unorganized stream of consciousness. A clinician has particular goals in mind when talking to clients, other professionals, or supervisors. For example, our goal might be to obtain specific kinds of information from a client or family member during a diagnostic interview. Obviously, it would help to have thought about the types of information you need and mentally prepare for the interview. Some clinicians make general notes regarding areas of discussion in the diagnostic interview. It is much better to be organized than to complete the interview and discover that you have not asked some important questions. Another example might be that you are asked to participate in a multidisciplinary staffing of your case with other professionals. Again, these other professionals do not have time to listen to a rambling, unorganized discussion of your dealings with the client. You should have your remarks outlined and any visual aids (e.g., handouts, treatment data) prepared prior to the staffing so that you can present a coherent description of your client. When talking with your clinical supervisor, it is always a good policy to organize your information prior to the meeting. If you are talking about treatment progress or you have questions for your supervisor, these can all be organized and discussed in a logical way rather than haphazardly. Thus, it is clear that verbal interactions with clients, other professionals, and supervisors are not mysterious and unpredictable. You should prepare for these meetings ahead of time by organizing what you will say. You might have to do this on paper in the beginning, but with more experience you will be able to mentally organize your discourse.

Use Professional Tone

You will recall that we introduced the notion of *professional tone words* in Chapter 8. By using these words, clinicians make their reports sound professional, and it is no different in verbal communication. The key in verbal interaction, however, is that the clinician must judge whether such terms would be appropriate for the person involved in the communication. For instance, if talking to a classroom teacher, a term such as *literacy* would probably be understood. Similarly, you might use the word *cognitive* when talking with a psychologist. On the other hand, if you were talking with a parent who had an eighth grade education, it would not be appropriate to use a term such as cognitive because he may not have been exposed to it. Thus, it is important to use professional tone words in verbal communication as much as possible, but you should always consider the background of the listener. While you may want to impress them with jargon from your academic classes, you should make your best attempt to speak in language that they will be able to process and understand. Define any jargon you use and attempt to personalize any suggestions to increase the likelihood of follow-through. After hearing the client's concerns, you may need to adjust your typical presentation of results to accommodate a higher or lower level of education, understanding and/or cultural differences. When the use of professional tone words may result in confusion, it is important to simplify your language, in order to communicate effectively.

Listen and Understand

Professional verbal communication is a two-way street. You are not talking with clients/family members, professionals, and supervisors just to hear the sound of your own voice. Thus, it is important to be a good listener when engaging in professional verbal communication. Most counseling texts suggest that it is critical that we listen to others for both the *content* and the *affect* of what they are saying (Crowe, 1997). The notion of content refers to the actual words and information that the person is providing. For instance, if a parent says, "Jeremy said his first word at age 3," the content would be the literal information provided by the mother. However, if the mother said the above utterance while a tear ran down her cheek and her voice broke in the middle of the sentence, this illustrates the affect or emotional tone of the utterance. Attending to both the content and affect of utterances in professional verbal interactions is very important. In the above illustration, we might want to engage the mother in further conversation about how she feels about her child's disorder. She may simply need to vent her concern and disappointment, or she may need a referral to a counselor if it seems like the feelings are affecting her life negatively. The point here is that we would not want to simply jot down that her child said his first word at age 3 and ignore the clear expression of emotion.

It is important to let your client know that you empathize and care about them and what they are going through. Haynes and Pindzola (2012) offer the following suggestions for the occasions when clients express emotion:

■ Avoid superficial statements of reassurance
■ Do not use terms or suggest consequences that will precipitate more stress for the client
■ Do not communicate any negative expectations regarding the outcome of therapy to the client

They additionally note that "the best antidote to fear and uncertainty is knowledge." This emphasizes the importance of your knowledge regarding their disorder and also your ability to effectively relay the details to them.

The same principle applies when dealing with other professionals. If you are trying to engage a classroom teacher to help with language stimulation for a preschool child and she says, "Sure, I'll help with the speech therapy; I don't have anything else to do," there is something more in that utterance than her willingness to assist in treatment. She is obviously feeling overwhelmed with her job and views your suggestions as an intrusion. If you attended to this emotional tone, you might indicate that you will be willing to come into the classroom and handle certain activities or assure the teacher that your suggestions can be implemented while she handles her regular routine.

The listening principle also applies to communicating with clinical supervisors. If you ask for therapy suggestions and your supervisor asks, "Have you looked in your class notes and in the library?" the real message is that you need to take more responsibility for coming up with ideas rather than being "spoon-fed" by your supervisor. Never underestimate the importance of not only *listening* but *understanding* your partners in verbal communication.

Attend to Context

Every verbal communication takes place in a context. The idea of communicative context has several components to which a professional must attend. Specifically, we are referring to (a) who you are talking to, (b) where you are talking, and (c) the feedback that you receive from your communication partner. First, you must consider the person to whom you are talking. This person possesses certain background knowledge, has a specific position in the social/professional hierarchy, and represents a unique cultural history. Any verbal communication must take into account these "who" variables whether you are speaking to clients/family members, other professionals, or your clinical supervisor. Let's say you are working with a Native American family from a lower socioeconomic level who has a child with a language disorder. You cannot assume that this family will inherently understand the nature, assessment, and treatment of child language disorders. Thus, your use of professional tone words will have to be reduced in favor of more "client-friendly" language. Several sources report that many cultures are not comfortable in revealing personal information to relative strangers (Battle, 1997; Roseberry-McKibbin, 1997). A good clinician will take this into account and perhaps postpone some of the more sensitive questioning until after a stronger relationship has been formed with the family. It is easy to see that appreciating the context of professional verbal

communication is an important variable in dealing with clients. It is also significant when dealing with other professionals. For example, when you talk to a classroom teacher, you can assume background knowledge about the educational milieu and the types of problems typically seen in SLP and teacher collaborations. You can use "educational" vocabulary and even some vocabulary specific to SLP if you have worked with this teacher before. If this teacher is also the principal of the school, she is treated with more respect and deference than a teacher with no administrative role in the school hierarchy. If the teacher is Hispanic, you want to make certain that you do not make any cultural gaffes in your conversation that might be offensive to a member of that ethnic group. Thus, the "who" of verbal communication partially defines how the conversation takes place.

The "where" of verbal communication also dictates the nature of a professional conversation. If you are talking in a hospital setting it is appropriate to use medical terminology shared by physicians, nurses, OTs, and PTs. You can assume that a term such as *FIM score* will be understood by most people you are working with. But, even though you are in a hospital, you must also remember the "who" factor. If you are talking to a family member of a teenager with a head injury, the term FIM score will be meaningless, and you have to modify your language to suit the listener. Similarly, when talking in an educational setting, you might assume that most teachers, special educators, and school psychologists share knowledge of certain terminology unless it is very discipline specific. At any rate, it is fine to throw around terms like *IEP* and *benchmark* with most educational personnel: just don't mention *diadochokinetic rate*.

Modify Based on Feedback

In any professional conversation with clients, professionals, and supervisors, there will be turn taking and interchange of both verbal and nonverbal communication. Sometimes, even if you have been respectful, organized your thoughts, used professional terminology, listened to content/affect, and attended to context, there will be miscommunication and error. This is why a professional always examines the nonverbal and verbal feedback from a conversational partner. If you are explaining the assessment results to parents and they begin to look quizzically at you, it is time to rephrase your utterance so that it can be understood. Parents or caregivers may be reluctant to ask you to repeat so it is vital that you are looking for cues that they do or do not understand what you are saying. If you are explaining your test results/ recommendations to a physician and he starts shaking his head, you will need to address any concerns that are present in your next utterance. Thus, it should be no surprise that professional verbal communication forms a feedback loop by which we constantly monitor our conversation and make changes to optimize communication. Ideally, we generate the optimal utterances on the initial attempt, but in cases where there is misunderstanding, we always have an opportunity to clarify.

THE VALUE OF EXPERIENCE

As we stated earlier, the critical elements discussed above are a part of any professional verbal communication, whether it is to clients, professionals, or supervisors. As a beginning student in clinical practicum you have no doubt marveled at the verbal ability of your supervisors in talking with parents, family members, and other professionals. How do they get to be so confident and able to think on their feet? Well, like many other enterprises, it all gets better with experience. As clinical supervisors, we understand that students typically feel underqualified and not equipped to evaluate, treat, and counsel adults as they are much younger than their clients or the caregivers they are interacting with. Be encouraged by the research of Haynes and Oratio (1978) that researched intervention effectiveness and found that adult clients value technical and interpersonal skills more than a clinician's age, gender or race. Therefore, acting in a professional and pleasant manner is more important to the client than the difference in age.

Most students feel completely inept when someone mentions the word "counseling." They frequently report that they don't feel competent in counseling another individual about anything, as the word counseling conjures up thoughts of delving into an individual's private life, using psychological lingo and worst of all, taking on the responsibility of someone else's problems. It's no wonder students shy away from any situation that might require they counsel their clients about their communication disorder. But, what we always tell students is that the way they become good at counseling, is to become as knowledgeable as possible about the client's disorder. Then, they are able to counsel their client based on knowledge, backed by research and clinical practice, not on conjecture. Most people appreciate someone being honest with them about whatever it is they are dealing with. And unfortunately, many people are never told exactly what their disorder is, what caused it, and what they can do to deal with it. That's what the competent, professional SLP is able to address when faced with issues that a client is dealing with regarding their disorder.

You will find that in the beginning of your practicum experience you will probably not be given assignments to talk with clients on your own. Instead, you will most likely sit in on sessions where your clinical supervisor carries out the interview or parent training or presents information at a staffing with other professionals. One reason why your opportunities at professional verbal communication will be severely limited at the beginning of practicum is that this is a skill that does not come naturally to any student. You first need to observe competent models of professional verbal communication from experienced clinicians. As you progress in clinical practicum, you will be trusted to take on more of the responsibilities of verbal communication with clients. By the time you are finishing graduate school, you will have seen many different styles of interaction with clients and their families. Ideally, you will be given opportunities to observe your supervisors in a variety of counseling situations so you can learn from them. You will then find yourself incorporating the styles of various supervisors with your own personality that will ultimately result in your own style of professional verbal communication. Before you graduate, you should have had the experience of conducting a variety of types of verbal communication with little supervision as you talk to clients, families, and other professionals.

CONTEXTS OF VERBAL COMMUNICATION WITH CLIENTS AND FAMILIES

There are at least six major contexts in which you will be using professional verbal communication with clients and families: (a) a diagnostic interview with parents of a child client; (b) a diagnostic interview with an adult client; (c) a diagnostic interview with the family of an adult client; (d) conducting training sessions for developing a home treatment program and/or their caregivers; (e) discussing treatment progress with clients and/or their caregivers; and (f) counseling clients and/or their caregivers about treatment issues. Within each of the aforementioned situations, you will be interviewing, providing informational counseling, providing personal adjustment counseling, or a combination of these. It is impossible to do justice to the field of counseling in a couple of short chapters. We refer you to other sources for a more detailed treatment of interviewing and counseling (Crowe, 1997; Emerick, 1969; Haynes & Pindzola, 2012; Shipley, 1997). We talk generically about dealing with clients in the six areas mentioned above. Although there are disorder-specific considerations for every type of communication impairment, there are also some general principles that can be applied to interviewing and counseling no matter what the disorder. We provide a brief sketch of some salient points from each area in the following sections.

INFORMATIONAL COUNSELING

Informational counseling is when you educate the client with information regarding the type and severity of the disorder, communication strengths and weaknesses, and your recommendations. You will be given the opportunity to provide informational counseling during both evaluation and treatment sessions. Informational counseling requires preparation. In a situation in which you know you are about to evaluate or treat a patient with a specific disorder with which you are not familiar, take time to research the characteristics of the disorder so that you have a better understanding of the possible nature of the patient's concerns. Even if you are familiar with the disorder, it may be a good idea to again familiarize yourself with norms and/or typical development so you can provide concrete examples of what is expected with regard to your client's age, gender, background and/or medical history. Sometimes clients have misconceptions about different aspects of evaluation, treatment, and prognosis and in researching the disorder prior to speaking with them, you will be able to dispel any myths they may believe.

After an evaluation or treatment session, it is appropriate to provide a summary to the client about your assessment of the client's performance, as well as strengths and weaknesses. Citing specific examples allows you to provide concrete and objective observations when discussing the client's communication. Of course, it is always preferable to begin with strengths and then move to detailing weaknesses.

When providing counseling after an evaluation session, the time in which you counsel a client or caregiver is dependent upon many variables and is not limited to the type and severity of the disorder, type and extent of testing administered, client knowledge of deficits, and individual needs. Counseling after treatment sessions is usually more brief, however, again varies on an individual basis and includes reference to performance and home program suggestions. Regardless of the situation, it is imperative that you allow the individual(s) a reasonable amount of time for information transfer and questions. You want to ensure they have understood the vital pieces of information that you are wishing to communicate.

Three Important Issues Common to All Diagnostic Interviews

We discuss some factors related to conducting diagnostic interviews with parents, family members, and adult clients in the next portions of this chapter. While it is beyond the scope of the present text to provide detailed coverage of how to conduct interviews for every disorder seen by the SLP, we first mention some important issues that are common to any diagnostic interview with any of the above groups.

The Interview Setting

Remember that one aspect of professionalism is the context in which clinical activity takes place. We want the interview room to be professional in appearance. This means it should be neat, clean, comfortable, and private. You must consider that the parents, client, or family members will be revealing personal information that should be kept confidential. This means that we do not perform a diagnostic interview in a waiting room or hallway. There should be some privacy provided for activities such as in an office or treatment/evaluation room.

Setting the Tone

A diagnostic interview is not simply a social chat. The interview is directed by the clinician, although the parents, client, or family members may not be aware that it is a directed conversation. It is up to the clinician to set the tone for the interview by telling the parents, client, or family members what will transpire (Matarazzo & Wiens, 1972; McQuire & Lorch, 1968). The box shows a brief example.

> Mr. and Mrs. Jones, I wanted to start by saying that I'm pleased to meet both of you and your son Brad. To begin, I want to let you know what we will be doing today for Brad's evaluation. First, I know that you have filled out our case history forms and I have read those before this meeting. During the first part of our meeting today I would like to clarify several things you mentioned in the paperwork and see if I can get some more information that will help me as we do the evaluation. So, first we will talk about Brad, and then I will be giving him some tests and taking some samples of his communication. After we are all finished with the assessment, we will meet with you again and let you know our preliminary findings and recommendations. At that time you might have questions that we can answer. It's better to save your questions for later on because we will be able to answer them more fully after seeing Brad. Right now, I would like to ask you some questions about Brad because you know him better than anyone else and can give me examples of what he is having difficulty with.

Notice how the clinician speaks formally, yet in a friendly manner. Note also that the clinician has sketched out how the evaluation will flow from obtaining information and assessing the child to providing information and making recommendations.

The Presenting Story

Most authorities on clinical interviewing suggest that clients come to the experience with a "presenting story" that they have rehearsed prior to the actual meeting (Emerick, 1969). You have no doubt experienced this yourself as a patient going to a physician for diagnosis of a medical problem. On your way to the doctor you might think about the types of symptoms you have been experiencing and what you have done to help yourself. Some people even talk through this presenting story in their car while driving to the doctor's office. It is important to let the patient reveal the presenting story because it contains his reason for coming into the clinic, his perception of the problem, and any misconceptions he might have regarding the situation. There are some ways to elicit the presenting story in the box.

> I'd like to begin by having you tell me what led up to your coming to the clinic for an evaluation.
>
> So, how can we help you with Brad?
>
> I know you've filled out our paperwork, but sometimes it is helpful to have you provide a little background in your own words about your concerns.
>
> I'd like to start by having you tell me about your concerns and why you came in today.

Notice how the clinician leaves it open-ended so that the parents can describe in detail their concerns and issues. These can be followed up by questions from the clinician when information is not clear. It is almost always good to ask parents for an example of behaviors they are concerned about. Sometimes clients, parents, or family members have misconceptions about their child's situation. We should always listen to these but not correct the client at this point in the interview. Later, when we provide information about the evaluation we can clarify any misconceptions that exist. For example, see the box.

In the diagnostic interview the mother says:

Brad mispronounces everything and people can't understand him. I've got this Uncle Calvin who is mentally retarded and nobody could understand him either. We hope that Brad isn't, you know, slow like Calvin.

After the evaluation the clinician says:

Earlier you mentioned a concern that Brad might be misarticulating because of mental retardation. First of all, most people with mental retardation who misarticulate have problems with vocabulary and sentence structure and show delays in many areas such as motor skills, social development, play, and activities of daily living. Brad has near-normal language and he has normal social, motor, and self-help skills. From Brad's language ability, his play, and the way he is interested in complicated videogames, I can tell you that he does not behave like a child with mental retardation. Research has shown that most children with misarticulations similar to Brad's are of normal or above intelligence. In his case we feel the problem is confined to speech sounds.

There are three classical parts to a diagnostic interview, whether it is with parents, clients, or family members. According to Haynes and Pindzola (2012), the interview is designed to do three things *in this order*: (a) obtain information, (b) provide information, and (c) provide counseling if necessary. Let us briefly go over these three components of a diagnostic interview as illustrated with parents.

Diagnostic Interview with Parents

One of the most important objectives of a diagnostic interview is to obtain information from the client/family. It is usually wise to focus on background information first to help you compensate for omissions and ambiguities in the case history. In many instances, responses on a case history form raise more questions than they answer. For instance, the parent might have indicated that the child takes a lot of medications, but has failed to mention what specific types of drugs are taken. You would want to follow up on this by saying, "In the case history you mentioned that your son takes several medications.

Can you tell us what they are?" Sometimes parents will say something very general or ambiguous that you would like a specific example of, such as, "Joey has behavior problems." There are many types of behaviors that are typical in children (e.g., tantrums) and those that are of more concern (e.g., lighting fires, abusing animals). It is always good to solicit examples from parents if they have been ambiguous. You can see that there can be many general issues to clarify in a diagnostic interview, and usually the initial part of the interview is spent disposing of these background issues. But we are not done obtaining information yet. Some writers have characterized the diagnostic interview as a "funnel" in which we begin talking about general information and then focus more tightly upon specific issues (Emerick, 1969; Stewart & Cash, 2010). Thus, we rarely go into a diagnostic evaluation of a child knowing nothing about the disorder of major concern to the family. Typically, we will have read case history forms that have been completed by the parents prior to the actual evaluation date or spoken with them over the phone. In most cases, the case history information will have a statement of the problem according to the parents, and this gives us a general guide to planning the evaluation. For instance, the parents might indicate that they are concerned about disfluencies, hoarseness, language development, or articulation errors. These statements of concern help us to focus the evaluation and the questions posed in the diagnostic interview. If the problem is hoarseness, you will want to ask questions about activities that could contribute to vocal abuse/misuse. You will also want to know how the vocal quality changes throughout the day, and if it had a sudden or gradual onset. There are many areas of questioning that are specific to each disorder of communication and you should be prepared to ask them in an evaluation.

As you are selecting standardized and nonstandardized measures to use in the evaluation session, you should also be thinking about questions you would like to ask the parents when they come for the assessment. Organization has been a common thread winding through this text, and you can see that it is important in conducting a parent interview. Beginning clinicians should write down areas of concern in which more information is needed. We do not suggest writing down *specific questions* because, as mentioned in a previous section, you do not know the parent's level of understanding. You could craft a specific question, and it might be too technical for some parents or not specific enough for others. Jotting down "areas" that you want to research is a more flexible approach. So, for example, if you have a concern about hearing loss and the parent has not addressed this in the case history, you should ask about hearing in the interview. The major point here is that you should never go into a parent interview unprepared. You should arrive at the interview with a legal pad that has specific issues written on it *in a logical sequence.* If you want to get more information on the biological foundations of communication, group your questions appropriately (e.g., hearing, motor skill, injuries, illnesses, medications). For example, do not skip from hearing to play to social friendships and then back to illnesses. Obviously, organization and planning of an interview can be done for any suspected area of concern in communication disorders whether it is language, phonology, fluency, or voice. You should look carefully at the case history information and then in your class notes and textbooks for specific background information that should be probed for the type of communication disorder of concern to the parents. Before the evaluation, it is a good idea to show your proposed interview protocol to your supervisor. We guarantee you that the supervisor will be impressed with a student who has thought about and planned a clinical interaction with parents.

We need to mention an important thing about the conduct of a diagnostic interview. The clinician is in control of this conversation and must direct it from the outset. Interviews are not the same thing as a social chat that moves randomly from topic to topic. You should set the tone for the interview by telling the family how it will proceed. You can indicate that the first part of the conversation will be to get information from the family because, after all, they are the most knowledgeable about their particular situation and concern. Once the parents know that you want information to use in your assessment, they usually cooperate by giving examples and answering your questions. Sometimes parents want to ask questions during the obtaining information portion of the interview (e.g., "What causes a child to have delayed speech?"). This is guaranteed to get you off the track of obtaining information and it is best to

stick to your plan. You might say, "I'll be able to answer you better after the evaluation when I've had a chance to see how Henry does on our tests. We'll have plenty of time to go over everything, but right now I want to learn about what you have done to help him at home." Once you have all the information you require, it is time to do the actual evaluation and gather data on the child's performance on standardized and nonstandardized tasks.

After the evaluation tasks, the parents will no doubt want to hear something about the results. No one wants to come to an evaluation and be told to go home without at least some preliminary information. Obviously, you will not have time to formally score all the standardized tests and transcribe/analyze a language sample on the day of the evaluation. You will, however, know some general pieces of information about the child's performance and be familiar enough with the case to know whether or not treatment is recommended. Thus, providing information can be conceived as having three parts. The first part of providing information is to summarize as many of the test results as you can, if only on a general level. Although you may not have scored a test, you will know that he missed a lot of items on certain subtests, or that he was able to complete other items without difficulty. You will know about language errors he made from a conversational sample. From your knowledge of normal communication development, you should know whether or not the child's performance is similar to other children at this age level. After summarizing the general test results, you then move toward interpreting the test results and talking about prognosis. The parents need to know what it means when you say that he performed poorly on an articulation test, but his performance on language tests was normal. For example, parents may not know that phonological and linguistic disorders are often co-occurring, but in Henry's case, his main difficulty is with the speech sounds. They also need to know that because he was stimulable, has normal hearing, has an interested family, and has no language problems, he has a good chance to perform well in therapy. After summarizing and interpreting the test results, you are ready to make recommendations. You might recommend treatment two times per week for 30 minutes for work on specific phonemes or phonological processes. The point here is that you have provided information in a systematic way moving from test results to interpretation to recommendation. Again, organization is key to professional verbal communication. The box gives an example of providing information to parents of a child who was evaluated for a fluency disorder. Notice that the clinician summarizes the test findings, and then moves into interpretation and finally into recommendations. Note also that the clinician leaves time for the parents to ask questions.

The Results

Well, we've finished all of our testing of Michael and I'd like to tell you what we found. First of all, Michael did fine on all of the language and articulation tests we administered, so he seems to be developing sentence structure, comprehension of language, and speech sounds in a normal fashion. He also has normal hearing according to our screening. We took a large conversational speech sample and we did notice various types of disfluencies in his speech. For example, he repeated whole words, phrases, parts of words, and some individual speech sounds when he talked. We also noticed some tense pauses in his speech where he abruptly stopped talking, breathing, and voicing. Another thing he did was to put filled pauses like "uh" in his sentences when he had trouble. He also showed some struggle behavior when he seemed to get stuck on a word.

Interpretation

So the language, hearing, and articulation results are very positive and we have no concern in those areas. In the area of fluency it is important to note that most children Michael's age repeat words and sentences as part of normal development and he has those kinds of repetitions in his speech. You mentioned earlier that you were concerned about the development of stuttering. Some of the things that suggest the possible development of a stuttering problem are things like repeating parts of words such as syllables, and repeating individual sounds such as "k-k-k-k-kite." Also, tense pauses and struggle behaviors are associated with the onset of stuttering in many children. You also mentioned in our earlier interview that Michael's uncle had a stuttering problem. If we look at all these things together, we feel that Michael is not merely producing normal developmental disfluency, but is showing some warning signs of continuing to stutter.

Recommendations and Prognosis

Because Michael is less than 4 years old we feel he has a good chance to become more fluent with therapy. Usually, the earlier a stuttering disorder is caught, the better the outlook. Also, because his language abilities are normal and his parents are concerned, he has a lot of positive things going for him. We would recommend that Michael come to therapy two times a week and that we work with you on some things that might help him be more fluent at home. Now, are there any questions you have for me?

The final component of the diagnostic interview is providing personal adjustment counseling, if necessary. In the vast majority of cases, no counseling issues arise in the diagnostic session. Sometimes, parents will react emotionally if they are hearing for the first time that their child really has a communication disorder. Perhaps they have been holding on to the hope that their child has normal speech and language abilities and just wanted to have that notion confirmed. Another issue might be concern over finances and if they can afford to pay for treatment. Most universities have sliding fee scales, or the parents can be referred to the public school system where treatment is free of charge. The point here is that if a parent expresses a real concern, emotional or not, you cannot just send him home to ruminate about it. If there is something you can say to ease the concern, you should do it. Again, in most cases this will not be necessary, but remember what we said in an earlier section about listening for content and affect in your clients.

Diagnostic Interviews with Adult Clients and Their Family Members

You will notice that we have combined the next two areas of professional verbal communication in dealing with clients and families. Mercifully, many of the same issues we raised in the previous section on diagnostic interviews with parents apply to these other groups. We are still conducting a professional interview and we still have our three goals of obtaining information and providing information and counseling, if needed. There are some slight differences in working with adult clients and their families. First of all, when interacting with parents, we are really not asking the young child questions during the interview. The parents are the most reliable informants for younger children. For older children, however, it is critical to involve them actively in the interview. For school-age children, you may choose to involve the child and a parent in the interview to get the most comprehensive information. In the case of adult clients, however, they can speak for themselves and should be allowed to do so unless they are incapacitated. For example, a client who has had a stroke and cannot talk would not be able to provide information during the evaluation. In that case, interviewing a family member is a reasonable method of obtaining this information. We must always be careful, however, to maintain the dignity and respect of the client. We do not want to talk about him as if he is not there. It is always good to involve the client in the interview, if for no other reason than to confirm what the family member has said. Some clinicians ask questions first of the patient, and then turn to the family member if he is unable to respond. Then you can ask the patient if that information is correct, or make a comment related to the new information. Even if you do not ask a question, you can let the patient know where you are going with the interview. For example, you might say, "I'd like to learn a little about the work that you did with the government. Is it all right if I ask your wife to tell me about that?" Again, you are still trying to obtain information from the client or family member, just as you would do when talking to parents. In most cases, adult clients are fully capable of speaking for themselves. Adults who stutter or have minor language problems, phonological disorders, or a vocal disorder can give you information directly during the diagnostic interview. For all adult clients, you must organize your questioning in a logical se-quence for the disorder area that is of concern to the client, just as we illustrated in the previous section on the parent interview. Obviously, with an adult client, your questions will revolve around vocational and daily obligations, rather than their performance in school and achievement of developmental milestones. The order of the diagnostic interview,

however, does not change. First you obtain information, and then you administer various diagnostic tests. After testing, you provide information about test results/ interpretation and make recommendations. If the client has major questions or concerns that require brief counseling, you provide it as needed. Margolis (2004) compiled the following suggestions based on numerous research studies to effectively communicate diagnostic recommendations and results.

Methods of Maximizing Retention

- In giving advice, use concrete instructions. "Say each word on this list, emphasizing the /f/ sound and ask your child to repeat" is more effective than, "Here is something to practice at home."
- Use easy-to-understand language, with short words and sentences.
- Present the most important information first (the primacy effect). Often, the most important information is a recommendation, such as, "make an appointment with the ear doctor."
- Stress the importance of recommendations or other information that you want the patient to remember.
- Use the method of explicit categorization. Tell the patient, "We are going to go over recommendations, then we will talk about your child's language problem (diagnosis), then we will go over test results, then we will talk about the plan of treatment and what you can do at home. (prognosis)." Ask for questions before moving on to the next category.
- Repeat the most important information.
- Don't present too much information. Present only what the patient needs to remember.
- Be sure you understand what clients want from the evaluation and what their beliefs are concerning the problem. Specifically address the patient's desires and beliefs.
- Supplement verbal information with written, graphical, and pictorial materials that the patient can take home.

Conducting Training Sessions for Developing a Home Treatment Program

In most treatment approaches that seek to improve speech and language, it is desirable to develop a home program to facilitate the generalization of communication skills learned in the clinic to other environments. Usually, the success of home programs depends to a large degree on the amount of direct training provided to the family and the clinician's ability to communicate what is to be done. Therefore, for a program to be successful there must be some type of organization in presenting the information to parents or clients. In child language, for example, Paul (2006) outlines many parent programs that take a structured approach to training for generalization to the home environment. In other words, for a home program to succeed, the parents or family members must be specifically trained to carry out the generalization activities. You are not establishing a home program when you walk the client down the hall after therapy and suggest they do a little of this and a little of that. Such suggestions, although not harmful, are not likely to be implemented correctly, or implemented at all, for that matter. On the other hand, if you use the last 10 minutes of your treatment session to invite the parent or family member into the therapy room and actually show him what to do and let him try it, that is a different story. This gives you the opportunity to critique the way he is performing the technique and provide reinforcement and suggestions. Our point here is that home programs can enhance generalization, but home programs are not as effective without specific training. This training is done through the use of professional verbal communication.

At times, we wonder why clients do not follow up on strategies or information we give them for use outside the therapy room. It may result from them not understanding what we said or being too embarrassed to not ask questions to clarify. Alternatively, they could be doing what they thought we said when that was not the suggestion at all. Fourie (2009) noted that adults with acquired communication disorders appreciate the SLP providing knowledge to them in terms that they can understand and providing practical and concrete suggestions.

The first step in training a parent or family member is to organize your training regime. There is that word again: organization. You must put some thought into what you want to train, the procedure to be used in training, and the most effective way to communicate this to the parent or family member. This is applicable to any type of training whether it is directed at language stimulation, reduction of vocal abuse, reacting to disfluency, or generalizing gains made in correct production of misarticulated phonemes. One important thing should be clear from the outset. We want the home program to involve fairly simple, straightforward, and doable tasks that can be easily fit into the daily routine. The parent should not be trained to do complex treatment tasks that are difficult to learn and carry out reliably. The general progression of such training has several components, no matter what the disorder area targeted. First, the clinician must tell the parent/family member about the general goals of the home program. If it is a child language case, it might be the use of recasting at home to facilitate generalization. Specifically, let's talk about a child who substitutes him/he and her/she. This child might say, "Her is my sister." We are working on the correct use of pronouns in clinical sessions, but we want to involve the parents in a home program to facilitate generalization. Much research has shown that recasting has been effective in training language across many different groups of children and a variety of language structures (Nelson, Camarata, Welsh, & Butkovsky, 1996). So, in this first step, we need to tell the parents that there is research that supports the use of recasting in language training and this is a technique that is fairly easy to learn and implement during daily interactions in the home environment. The clinician might define recasting as restating the child's incorrect utterance in a correct manner. For example, if the child says, "Her is my sister," the parent should say, "Yes, she is your sister." Recasts can easily be woven into conversations and they do not require the child to imitate or correct the utterance. All they do is immediately give the child a correct model of a sentence that he has produced incorrectly.

After outlining the technique that you want the parents to use, you move on to step two. In the second step of parent training, you actually demonstrate the technique with the child in the therapy room with the parent watching. In this way, the parent can see the procedure in action and it is not simply an abstraction that was talked about in step one. After several demonstrations, you move on to step three. In the third step, the parent is encouraged to try the technique with the child and the clinician provides feedback about effective use of the technique and anything that might be changed to make it more productive. In the fourth step, the parent is asked about situations in the home environment where recasting might be used. For instance, the parent might say that a lot of conversations with the child occur in the car when running errands and going to various sports practice events. This is a good time to have conversation and use recasts. Finally, the parent is asked to make some mental notes about the child's correct production of the target language structure. That is, we want the parent to notice if the child is beginning to use the correct forms more often.

It is clear that training parents/family members to do any type of home program is done by professional verbal communication. We explain, model, monitor, and charge the parent/family member with the responsibility of implementing the technique. This applies to everything from articulation disorders to vocal abuse to stuttering. The key is that the training is organized and professionally done by the clinician.

Discussing Treatment Progress with Clients and Families

It is the responsibility of any competent clinician to provide feedback to clients about how they are making progress in treatment. Ideally, this is done by presenting behavioral data showing that performance has changed over time. Again, this is accomplished using professional verbal communication. Certainly, you can give copies of treatment reports to clients/family members, but in most cases such reports are written in terms that are more appropriate for SLPs and other professionals. It is always a good policy to sit down with clients/family members and take stock of progress or lack thereof. In the university clinic, for example, the end of the semester is a good time to have such a conference. In the medical setting, you may be called upon for a brief report whenever a family member's visit overlaps with your therapy session.

As in any professional verbal communication, organization is again a central issue. You should not sit down with clients to casually discuss clinical progress without adequate preparation. Some obvious components of that preparation would be the data gathered throughout the semester, and in most cases it is good to display the data on a chart or graph. If the graph shows an increase in performance of treatment targets or a decrease in errors, most parents are satisfied that they are getting their money's worth. When explaining treatment progress, it is a good idea to recap the goals targeted in therapy and how they relate to the data presented. Another part of a treatment progress conference is to talk about the next set of goals that will be targeted in the next semester and ask for feedback from the parent or client. Although we all would like to make progress in treatment, there are cases in which the conference will demonstrate a decided lack of progress. If the graph is not moving away from baseline levels, then the discussion with the parents might focus on variables that need to be changed in order for progress to occur. For instance, a child who comes to treatment once a week for 30 minutes and is not making progress might need to try coming twice a week in order to have a positive response. Again, the data you present will support your suggestion. Do not forget to solicit client feedback in these progress conferences. Are there things they are especially pleased with regarding the treatment? Are there aspects of the therapy they do not understand? Do they have any concerns or issues they would like to raise? All of this is done using professional verbal communication and it is a critical component of a good clinical relationship with clients or families.

Counseling Clients and Families About Treatment Issues

On a realistic level, counseling in a clinical relationship is designed to solve problems and/or deal with feelings related to the treatment regime. Many types of problems may be associated with treatment such as irregular attendance to therapy sessions, lack of progress, unrealistic expectations on the part of the client/family, feelings of hostility or discouragement related to the treatment, lack of motivation, explaining changes in the treatment approach, transition to another service provider, or referral to a professional from a related discipline (e.g., psychology). Actually, the issues listed above might very well account for most of the counseling efforts in treatment encountered by students in clinical practicum, but there are certainly others we have not raised. While you may only not have a long history with the client, you will have to deal with the day-to-day occurrences that happen in the therapeutic relationship. Thus, it is the goal of this section to provide a *general* view of the process of communicating about counseling issues rather than an all-encompassing set of guidelines. For more detailed coverage of counseling we direct you to other sources (Crowe, 1997; Shipley, 1997).

Figure 9–2 shows a very basic process of identifying and dealing with treatment issues using profes-

sional verbal communication. This is fundamentally "problem solving;" however, you will see that confronting problems in clinical work often leads to talking about feelings and perceptions that are more sensitive than a simple social conversation. Thus, the approach we are taking to counseling is a series of steps for addressing problems that arise with clients in your practicum experience. We briefly discuss each step below, and guess what? Organization is a major factor in counseling, just as in every other aspect of professional verbal and written communication.

The first step in counseling about treatment issues is to identify the problem. In some cases, the client will be the person who identifies an issue of

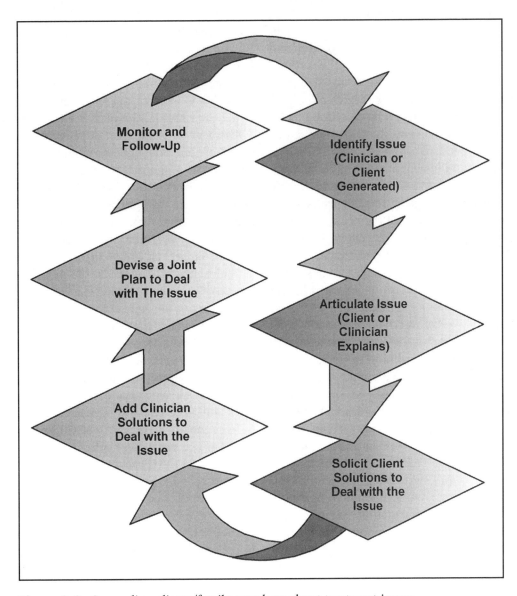

Figure 9–2. Counseling clients/family members about treatment issues.

concern. For example, after a treatment session one day, a client might express dissatisfaction with the amount of progress being made in therapy. Your first reaction might be to act defensive about such a comment and you might feel bad about your performance as a clinician. A positive aspect of this comment is that the client has brought it out into the open and has not internalized it and simply sabotaged the treatment by not trying or failing to attend therapy sessions. A good clinician simply cannot let this comment go by and not deal with it. Thus, we have a situation in which a client has identified an issue (dissatisfaction with treatment progress) and the clinician must find a way to explore the problem and suggest solutions. The second step in this process is to obtain the client's perception of the problem. Typically, the clinician can act as a facilitator to gain more insight into the issue. For instance, the clinician might say, "Let's talk about this for a while. Tell me some specific things that you are not satisfied with in our treatment approach or your progress. Then we can make some adjustments to the therapy or talk about your progress and how we can improve our approach." This opens up a "can of worms," but you can clearly see that allowing a client to go through the motions in treatment sessions while harboring such feelings is not productive. In some cases, there is simply a misunderstanding of the goals or unrealistic expectations on the part of the client. These can easily be dealt with by counseling the client on the difficulty of treatment and providing examples of the range of progress made by many clients working on the same type of communication disorder.

Sometimes there is a very specific issue that is bothering the client. For example, a client who stutters might be frustrated with clinical exercises involving easy onset and slowed speech rate because no generalization to daily situations is seen where the stuttering still occurs. Again, this can be dealt with by further explanation of the techniques, or more realistic situations can be integrated into the treatment in which the techniques can be used to facilitate fluency in everyday communication. Whatever the situation, it is always better to address it than ignore it.

After identifying the issue and articulating it, the focus should be on potential solutions to the problem. If you have not learned this already as part of your life, solutions are generally better when arrived at jointly by the people experiencing the problem. It is a wise clinician who solicits client solutions to a problem and then suggests some additional solutions to the mix. So we ask the client, "What do you think we can do to make better progress?" In some cases the client may say that more treatment sessions are needed. In other cases, the client may feel the clinician is not being aggressive enough in treatment. Other cases may want some different aspects added to the treatment approach. The next step is for the clinician to add possible solutions to those that the client has provided. Be sure to reinforce the client's suggestions if they are reasonable. "I really like your suggestion of using more realistic situations in therapy. Actually, I've got a whole file of real-life activities that we can arrange in order of difficulty and start using next week if you like."

So both the client and clinician have made positive suggestions for the treatment approach and the next step is to agree on a joint plan of action. If the client likes some of the ideas that were generated in joint discussion, the plan needs to be formalized. "Okay, it sounds like we are in agreement about the problem and some potential things to try in order to solve it. I'll bring my list of activities on Monday and we can prioritize them so we can work toward you being able to use your techniques in more realistic situations." Now, it might occur to you that the client may not be ready to produce fluent speech in more difficult situations. What if the person fails at the new activities? This is not all bad, because it may just be the dose of reality the client needed to justify more work on easy onset and slower rate in the clinic. All the counseling in the world may not make the client feel good about boring clinical activities, but experiencing difficulty on higher level tasks might bring home the realization that a bit more practice on the easy onset and slower rate is not such a dreadful idea after all. If the client is successful at more difficult tasks, it merely shows what a good clinician you are because you have responded to client suggestions that allowed faster treatment progress. If the client is not successful, again you have been responsive to concerns, but you were correct in your initial judgment of client abilities, and it is now clear why you started at that level.

The final step in the process is to monitor how the plan has worked. After trying out the plan agreed upon by the client and clinician, it is always a good idea to take stock of how things are going. "Well, we've tried some more realistic activities and you seem to be responding well according to our data on your disfluencies. How do you feel about your progress in therapy now?" This gives you an opportunity to attain closure on a problem that has been solved, and it also opens the door to making adjustment in the treatment that will fine-tune the approach.

Remember that we said the counseling issue might be raised by either the client or the clinician. For instance, the clinician may be concerned about the client's attendance, the inconsistent use of practice outside the clinic, or the lack of motivation. Any of these issues can and should be raised if they are on the clinician's mind. "We have you scheduled for therapy three times a week, and yet you are only coming one or two times. I'm afraid that this might be having an impact on your progress. There are a lot of reasons why people come inconsistently ranging from scheduling to money to transportation to motivation. So, tell me about why you are having trouble getting here and maybe we can come up with a plan to make things better." Again, you could just let it slide and not say anything, but you are not dealing with the underlying problem. Opening the door to discussing such issues is much better than ignoring them and hypothesizing all sorts of reasons that may not be true. Whoever raises the issue, client or clinician, the important thing is that the concern receives your attention. These concerns are dealt with exclusively using professional verbal communication as you identify issues, articulate them, solicit joint solutions, devise a cooperative plan, and monitor the plan to determine if it was or was not successful.

PERSONAL ADJUSTMENT COUNSELING

Fourie (2009) notes that SLPs need to be ready not only to treat the communication impairment itself, but also the issue of the impact of the communication disorder on the client. This type of counseling encompasses being available to assist your client in coping with the information you have provided.

Dependent upon your setting, you may encounter a person who has experienced a life change such as a stroke, diagnosis of head and neck cancer, or the recent diagnosis of a child with autism or cerebral palsy. They may be experiencing grief, anxiety, shock, frustration, or anger and you should be ready to listen when they share their concerns. Ignoring their concerns or changing the subject will communicate to your client that you are either disinterested or do not approve of what they are feeling. Kaderavek, Laux, and Mills (2004) found that the clinical counseling relationship significantly influences positive client outcomes. Therefore, if you don't effectively address your client's needs and concerns, their progress may be hindered with regard to therapy goals.

We would like to be clear at the outset: Counseling a client is serious business that takes years of training and experience to perform well. Just to give you some insight, Crowe (1997) discusses some of the following counseling opportunities that arise in SLP, depending on the client's age and type of disorder: (a) feelings of anxiety, grief, guilt, isolation, and anger; (b) denial of the problem; (c) dealing with a guarded prognosis; (d) self-concept; (e) cultural barriers; and (f) inaccurate perceptions and nonproductive attitudes. Shipley (1997) raises the specter of clients who are paranoid, overprotective, talk too much, are depressed, and may even contemplate suicide due to the changes in their lives after a stroke, laryngectomy, or degenerative neurological disease. Obviously, we do not expect students in training to delve into the psyches of their clients and deal with these major emotional and life issues. In some cases, even the experienced SLP must refer such seriously involved clients to professional counselors or psychotherapists. Most of the time we can deal with clients having a bad day by just being human, listening to them, and demonstrating that we understand their feelings. No one who is feeling depressed wants another person to deny the validity of his feelings and pretend that everything is all sweetness and light. Clients who become frustrated and depressed about their abilities after a stroke might say, "I used to be able to do woodworking in my workshop, but since the stroke, I can't use my tools. That was my favorite hobby and now I can't do it." A validation of their concern would be an appropriate response, such as, "I know how much you loved woodworking and it must be very frustrating not to be able to do that anymore." Remember the content and affect concept. In most cases, for practicum students, there are more basic issues to deal with that involve professional verbal communication. If serious counseling issues come up, the student needs to (a) recognize the issue, (b) address it if it is a fairly simple and straightforward problem, and (c) alert the clinical supervisor if the problem seems beyond his ability to deal with. It is always better to err on the side of caution rather than dabble in issues you are not equipped to handle. Your own experience will be a guide as well. For example, once you have counseled parents on children's behavior problems with the help of your supervisor, you should feel some confidence in addressing similar issues with a new case. On the other hand, if your client with a laryngectomy says she has no friends and does not want to live, you probably need to get some help from your supervisor.

It is tempting to want to focus specifically on your client's speech and language issues, but you must learn to view the client as a whole person, with needs in areas outside their communication skills. The focus should be on the client and his needs, rather than on you and the agenda you have for the evaluation or treatment session. According to Kaderavek, Laux, and Mills (2004), "This process includes learning to tolerate silence during the client-clinician interaction, to reflect client emotions, and to clarify clients' self-perceptions." Luterman (2001) noted that "clients' self-discovery and self-actualization is best accomplished by listening instead of prescribing." Moments of silence should not be feared but welcomed as a means of encouraging the client to continue speaking and to process information that you have communicated to them.

During treatment sessions, you may be forced to modify your plans based on the client's demeanor and level of motivation for that day. Therefore, it is pertinent that you take your lead from the client, and that you listen to them so you know how best to provide information and emotional support. Hackney and Cormier (1994), noted that the use of minimal encouragers, such as "mmm-hmm," "yes," or "I see" communicated the attention and approval of the clinician. Another aspect to consider is what you are communicating to the client through your nonverbal behavior. Appropriate facial expressions, deliberate head nodding, and a relaxed and slightly forward body position is regarded as indicating favorable affect and encouraging the client to speak more (Kaderavek, Laux, & Mills, 2004; Mehrabian, 1972; Shipley, 1997).

At the same time, you do not want to abandon therapy goals while the patient spends the entire session lamenting his troubles. Davis (2000), as cited in Fourie (2011, p. 58) gives advice for this. "On some days a patient may just want to talk, and a clinician may want to be sympathetic to the client's desire. However, the clinician has to make a judgment as to whether listening for a while is necessary for achieving successful stimulation on that day. The patient may need to vent, which should clear the air to resume treatment. In general, the clinician needs to manage valuable treatment time by gently steering the patient into planned activities." When listening and then responding to your client's concerns, you can reassure them by remaining calm and collected while problem solving with them regarding the issues related to their communication disorder.

The degree to which you serve as counselor varies according to the individual, their disorder, cultural background and issues stemming from their disorder or other life issues. It is vital for you as a professional to be ready to provide all types of counseling, as necessary for you to establish and maintain rapport with your client and/or their families. That being said, it may become apparent during your sessions that your patient could benefit from formal psychological services. It is your responsibility to address this need with your client and provide recommendations regarding possible resources and referrals. As cited in Atkins (2007, p. 5), ASHA stated that SLPs should "support their client's emotional and psychological concerns as they relate to the communication disorder." While it may be necessary to provide support in dealing with issues resulting from their communication disorder, it is not within the SLP's scope of practice to engage in formal psychotherapy. Although you may feel that you know exactly what course of action the client should take, avoid trying to solve the client's problems. Counseling a client is quite different than counseling a personal friend, and this requires awareness on your part to respond in an appropriate manner.

Scenario 1

You are in the middle of a diagnostic session with a client who has recently had a stroke. Your supervisor has told you to administer the *Boston Diagnostic Aphasia Examination*, and emphasized how important it is to complete the test for treatment planning purposes. After completing only two subtests, your client suddenly begins to tell you how upset he is about his inability to drive, and he begins crying and states that he does not want to be a burden on his family. What do you do? Although you may be tempted to avoid the issue and continue with the test, it is necessary and appropriate to stop and listen to what he is saying. Allow him to express his concerns, using empathy and good listening skills. If your client is given the opportunity to express his emotions in a nonjudgmental and supporting environment, you are on your way to establishing trust and rapport. More than likely, you will be able to continue the assessment with your client less distracted and able to persevere with genuine effort. If the concern is related to an allied professional (in this case an Occupational Therapist), make that referral, or if necessary, to a counselor or psychologist.

Scenario 2

You have been working with a 2-year-old client for approximately 5 weeks. Your client is nonverbal and demonstrating behaviors that are consistent with Autism Spectrum Disorder, although he has not been diagnosed. At this time, he has been diagnosed with a receptive and expressive language delay, and possibly PDD. One day, your supervisor is away from the clinic at a conference, and your client is avoiding eye contact and exhibiting various types of self-stimulating behavior. The parent comes up to you after the session and asks, "Do you think my child has Autism?" What do you do? Even though you are not qualified to make this diagnosis, you are able to say to the parent, "I understand your concerns, and based on what I've learned in my classes, I have seen some behaviors that are common in children on the spectrum. Next week, my supervisor will be back, and I will arrange for her to discuss this with you prior to the session. It may be necessary for us to make a referral for your son to be evaluated by another professional who could do additional testing prior to a diagnosis."

This chapter aimed to illustrate some basic principles of professional verbal communication with clients and families. As a student in clinical practicum, you will do far more communicating verbally than on paper with your clients and family members. This verbal communication is a platform by which you obtain information, provide information, and deal with problems that arise in the course of your clinical relationship. Always remember to be respectful, organized, professional in your language, a good listener, and attend to the context of communication so that your utterances will be appropriate in terms of the environment and the client's knowledge base and culture. If you remember these things when communicating verbally you will be perceived as a professional. Also, know that problems are bound to arise in any clinical relationship. It is always best to deal with such issues earlier rather than later. Whether the client raises the issue or you must bring up a sensitive problem, these concerns can be dealt with in a systematic way using professional verbal communication. The problem must be identified and discussed. A joint plan of action must be devised using input from both clinician and client. Finally, a mechanism to monitor whether or not the problem has been solved must be put into place. Throughout your career, you will be called upon to provide counseling to persons of all ages with various cultural, educational, cognitive, and socioeconomic backgrounds. Remember that it is your job to respectfully provide them with clear, pertinent and accurate information related to their communication disorder and specific strategies to increase their communication skills in their daily activities. Also, it is not your job as clinician to "cheer them up," but to empathize with them and then assist them in identifying possible solutions. Such problem solving is always a challenge, but it is a natural part of clinical responsibility, interaction, and ultimately success.

10 Interacting with Other Professionals

In the beginning of your clinical practicum experience you will probably have little opportunity to directly interact with other professionals. This is because initial practicum assignments are typically in the university clinic. Usually such clinics are staffed solely by speech-language pathologists and audiologists, unless the clinic operates in tandem with other departments on campus such as special education, psychology, or health professions. Although such models exist on university campuses, they are not the norm. As you progress in your practicum experience, you will find yourself interacting with more professionals from other disciplines as you are assigned to rehabilitation centers, hospitals, schools, or long-term care facilities. Even in the beginning, however, you might have the opportunity to collaborate with other professionals on a case you are working within the university clinic. For example, you may be working with a child who has a language/phonological disorder. It is possible that this child is attending public school and is also receiving treatment from the school SLP. This child will also have a classroom teacher and may be receiving other services from a specialist in learning disabilities. Thus, even though your work is confined to the university clinic you might come in contact with these other professionals for a variety of reasons. First, you might be interested to know about the IEP goals that your client is working on in the public schools. To find this out, you have to contact the school SLP either in person, by telephone, by e-mail, or by letter to obtain the relevant information. A second reason to contact the public school professionals is to determine how your approach at the university could make the best contribution to the child's overall treatment regimen by coordinating your goals with those of the school personnel. For instance, they might be working on literacy issues and grammar but have little time to work on phonology and pragmatics. The university program could coordinate work on a variety of goals so that some are not ignored or duplicated across settings. This coordination takes professional verbal communication. A third reason to contact the school professionals is to determine how the work you are doing with the child in the university clinic is generalizing to the school environment. You may want to visit the school and observe your client's communication in the academic setting. During this visit, you will no doubt come in contact with professionals who work in the school system. A final reason to contact the school personnel is to determine what curricular materials might be used in your therapy to result in maximum generalization. Most authorities in school-age language disorders suggest that treatment activities incorporate some curricular material such as grade or subject-specific vocabulary and discussion topics so that the child can receive an academic payoff in addition to the communicative gains.

Depending on the type of case, there may be other professionals dealing with your client simultaneously. Some campuses, for instance, have programs for children with autism. In such programs, the child may be seen in a preschool program in the department of special education or psychology and you might be doing your treatment either in the university clinic or in these other departments. Either way, you are in a position to interact with other professionals. Thus, you can see that interaction with other professionals can take place even when you are operating in the sheltered environment of the university clinic. As we said above, such interactions will only increase as your practicum experiences take you to other settings throughout graduate school.

In Chapter 9 we outlined several critical elements that should be part of professional verbal communication with clients and families. These elements were showing respect, organization, use of a professional tone, listening/understanding, and attending to the communicative context. All of these elements, crucial to interacting with clients/families, are just as important when dealing with other professionals. We gave several examples of how these factors apply to our conversations with professionals in Chapter 9. We just wanted to bring them back to a conscious level for the present chapter. It is assumed that you will attend to these critical elements of interaction in all your communications with professionals from other disciplines.

CONTEXTS OF VERBAL COMMUNICATION WITH OTHER PROFESSIONALS

There are at least four contexts in which you will be likely to interact with professionals from other disciplines: (a) consultations, (b) staffings/meetings, (c) collaboration, and (d) solving problems in informal daily interactions. We discuss each of these below to give you a flavor for how they unfold.

Consultations

In most instances the purpose of a consultation is to access additional information or a different perspective on your client. There are several reasons why the SLP will consult another professional about a case. In the first instance, you might want to consult a professional to obtain information that will assist you in your treatment program. We mentioned above a situation in which you might want to obtain information about the school curriculum and/or goals that the school SLP is targeting in treatment. In most cases, to be done effectively, this necessitates a face-to-face meeting. It is difficult to cover all the information over the telephone or in written communication, the latter of which does not allow for questions and clarification. A second reason to consult another professional is to ask for help that is discipline specific. For

instance, in working with a child who has autism you might have questions about how to deal with behavior problems that occur in treatment. In your search for answers you might ask a person from the psychology department to consult on the case. During this consultation, you could meet with the psychologist to discuss your concerns either in the psychology department or in the speech and hearing clinic. You might want to ask the psychologist to observe the child and provide suggestions on dealing with behavioral issues. As you progress in practicum to other work settings, it is not unusual to ask other professionals such as physical therapists, occupational therapists, nurses, or physicians for a formal or informal consult on a patient you are working with. Remember, there is a difference between an informal consultation and a formal referral for an evaluation by another professional. Informal consultations are usually a professional courtesy given to one person by another. Formal referrals for evaluation are done on a fee basis and often need doctor's orders or other administrative paperwork to occur. It is one thing to refer a child for a psychological evaluation, and quite another to ask for "input" from a colleague who works in your organization. As mentioned in Chapter 3, it is crucial to obtain a signed release of information from the client/parent before involving another professional in order to protect client confidentiality. Never underestimate the importance of obtaining a release of information before *any* consultation is done. Assuming we have permission, we might find the SLP asking the occupational therapist or physical therapist about positioning issues when working with a client who has motoric disorders. Because these other professionals are working with the client on activities of daily living, they are usually more than happy to give suggestions about positioning the client for activities involving the SLP. Similarly, other professionals will ask the SLP about the communicative status of a patient with whom they are both working and how best to have successful interactions. Such informal consults are part of working together as a rehabilitation team.

When asking another professional for a consultation, it is important to remember that you are requesting a favor. Thus, you can see why showing respect, organizing your request, talking professionally, listening carefully, and attending to context are critical. The box illustrates an example with a psychologist:

Telephone Contact

Hello Dr. Jarvis, this is Madeline Smith and I'm a speech-language pathology student working in the university speech and hearing clinic. My clinical supervisor suggested that I contact you about a child I'm working with on language development. The child has autism and is exhibiting some behaviors that we are having difficulty dealing with. I was wondering if it would be possible to set up a short meeting with you to get your input on what I might do to make my treatment more effective?

The Meeting

Thank you so much for taking the time to talk with me about Kevin. I would greatly appreciate any insight you might provide in this case. So I don't take up too much of your time, I've brought along some video examples of the behaviors I am having trouble with, so if you look at my camcorder screen you can see what I'm talking about. I'm especially concerned when Kevin hits and spits during therapy like in these examples. Right now, I'm dealing with this by telling him "No" when he does these behaviors, but it doesn't seem to reduce their occurrence. Do you have any suggestions?

Notice how the clinician called to set up the appointment to see if the psychologist was willing to consult. Also, note that the clinician got right to the point, showed the psychologist what she had concerns about, and indicated her current approach in dealing with the behavior. You can see that organization was important in obtaining this consultation. There was preparation time in terms of looking up the correct telephone number, making an appointment, selecting video examples of the behavior that was of concern, and telling the psychologist how the behaviors are currently being handled. After the meeting, it should go without saying that the clinician thanks the psychologist for the consult. It is always a nice touch to give feedback to the other professional, especially if her suggestion has been implemented and it was effective. Everyone likes to hear that her advice was followed and helped the situation. Also, it never hurts to let the other profes-

sional know that "if there is ever anything we can do for you on a case in the future please let us know." The box gives an example in a school system of consulting with a teacher:

Initial Contact in the Hallway

Hi, Mrs. Johnson, I was wondering if I could get some advice on Lester Hollis. Because you are his teacher and know how he responds, I'd like your input on combining some classroom material into his language goals. If you are willing, I'd be happy to come to your classroom after school some day for a few minutes to get your opinion on what I'm doing to incorporate the curriculum into his therapy.

The Meeting

Thank you so much for meeting with me about Lester. I've brought the materials I'm using with him and I wanted to show you how we are trying to incorporate American government into our language goals. You can see that I've made up an organizational chart we can use when we discuss how the government works to make laws. I was wondering if there are any other important government processes Lester and I can discuss in therapy that would also help him in the classroom.

Notice how the clinician approaches the teacher in a respectful manner and makes a convenient time to talk about the student. At the meeting, the clinician is well prepared and organized and asks specific questions about how to apply classroom work to treatment.

Consultation is an important component of the relationship between various disciplines. As your career progresses, you should be prepared to both request consultation from and provide consultation to other professionals. Verbal communication is the major vehicle for consultation, and for success to occur, it must be done in a professional manner.

Staffings and Meetings

In many work settings there is often the opportunity to "staff" a case that has common interest to a variety of professionals. Staffings usually focus on pulling together multidisciplinary assessment information from a variety of professionals, or they concern progress reports on a client who has been in treatment for a period of time. The two environments where staffings are most common are medical facilities and school systems. In some university clinics, students are asked to meet for the purpose of discussing their cases as part of a "grand rounds" experience or merely a case presentation. Such experiences in the university clinic give the beginning student a chance to organize and cogently present information on a client to faculty and peers in the training program. Presumably, it prepares these students for presentations they might have to make in other work settings later in their practicum experience. For example, in school systems there are IEP meetings and other opportunities to discuss the progress of students receiving therapy. In medical facilities, staffings are common and are attended by representatives of all health professions involved with the patient. Often, these staffings are weekly, or even daily, especially in facilities where the patient is staying for a limited time frame.

The conduct of a staffing is much like any meeting where there is an agenda. The purpose of the staffing is for all of the professionals who work with the patient to update the team regarding progress toward goals and any difficulties that may have arisen since the last meeting. Typically, one professional (and it could be from any discipline) directs the meeting. For example, in dealing with children, this person is often called the *case manager* and will facilitate the conduct of a staffing in which a child's treatment progress is discussed by the educational team. In some facilities the staffing concerns many patients, each of whom must be talked about by all relevant professionals. In these types of staffings, time is of the essence and each professional is allotted only a few minutes to report on the patient's progress. Thus, you will only have a short period of time to let the other professionals know how a particular patient is progressing toward goals. This is one reason why FIM scores are commonly used in medical facilities. It does not take long to report that "Mr. Jones has moved from a level X to a level Y on language comprehension." In other settings, however, the meeting or staffing concerns only a single client. For instance, there are clinics that provide in-depth multidisciplinary evaluations, and the purpose of the staffing is for each professional to provide detailed information on her assessment and finally to engage in a discussion of the combined results to arrive at treatment recommendations. Obviously, in this type of meeting you will have the floor for a longer period of time and go into significantly more detail. In some medical settings, difficult and complicated cases are staffed in detail with lengthy presentations by different professionals and a group discussion of recommendations.

If you are scheduled to participate in a staffing of your client next week, there are several things you should do in preparation. First of all, you should find out the nature of the staffing in terms of time allotted to each participant. It makes a great deal of difference if you have to prepare a 5-minute presentation or a 30-minute case summary. For our purposes, let's assume that you are scheduled to talk for 15 minutes about your case and the progress he has made in treatment over the last 3 months. If you have read this textbook thus far, you already know that merely showing up at the staffing with no preparation is not an option. Organization and preparation give you the opportunity to make a successful and informative presentation. Lack of preparation will result in a poor to mediocre presentation that will not reflect positively on you or the facility you represent.

After finding out the type of meeting you will be attending, you should assemble all of your data on the client so you can determine the information that will be the most relevant. In this particular case, you are charged with presenting information on the client's progress over a 3-month period. Thus, you probably will want to spend most of your presentation time on this topic rather than an extensive reiteration of the client's case history or his status 6 months ago. Although it is certainly acceptable to mention some historical information and intake data, your focus should be on the past 3 months. In many cases the same professionals sitting around the table will have attended a meeting on this same client 3 months ago when you talked about earlier therapy progress. In this case, they are familiar with background information and how the client first responded when entering the facility. So how do you prepare yourself to present the treatment progress over the last 3 months? A logical place to start is to mention all of the goals you were working on during that period. This can be followed by the presentation of treatment data on each goal, perhaps supported by graphs or handouts. The final portion of your presentation might focus on eliminating goals that have been accomplished and the establishment of new goals to be targeted in the next 3 months. Notice that the presentation is organized, focused, and packaged to fit into the time allotted. It is also important to remember that you must take into account your audience when you are presenting information at a staffing. Although you can use professional terms that cross disciplines, any concepts unique to SLP should be explained in easy to understand language to avoid confusion.

If you are not the first one to present, it is often useful to refer to the presentations of others to validate points you need to make in your summary. For example, if the occupational therapist reports that the patient has difficulty paying attention while learning self-help tasks, you might say, "Just as OT indicated, I have also noticed attention difficulties during my language treatment tasks." It not only shows that you are listening, but it validates the observation of someone else on the team and helps to consolidate information on the patient.

Staffings are not just serial reports by representatives of varied disciplines. Subsequent to individual reports, there is usually discussion centered on trying to integrate the reports and modify future goals based on client progress. Often, the discussion turns to problem solving in difficult cases. An important thing to remember is that you are part of a team that must reach some sort of consensus. You must strike a balance between raising issues and solutions you feel are important and allowing others to do the same. Staffings in which professionals provide no input and those in which a person dominates the group are equally unproductive. Remember, the client is the most important consideration in any staffing.

Staffings are an important part of working as an SLP. They should never be taken lightly because you are not only representing yourself and your facility, but the entire profession of speech-language pathology as well. Staffings are accomplished almost exclusively with verbal communication among professionals, so students should take advantage of the opportunity to watch supervisors and graduate students perform in this arena.

Collaboration

For years, SLPs have cooperated with professionals from other disciplines in what has become known as a *consultative model* or *collaborative model* of treatment. In these models, professionals from varied disciplines work together to facilitate treatment progress in a particular client. Haynes, Moran, and Pindzola (2006) outline collaborative models in terms of interdisciplinary, multidisciplinary, and transdisciplinary approaches to therapy. Each of these approaches involves members of various disciplines, but the interaction among the professions is quite different. In multidisciplinary approaches, for example, each profession sees the client separately and there is very little cross-disciplinary planning. There are separate and discipline-specific evaluations, goals, treatments, billing, and parent/family conferences. As mentioned above, a staffing may occur at some point, but it is usually discipline specific. A multidisciplinary staffing would consist of each discipline presenting what it did for the client and the progress achieved on targeted goals.

Interdisciplinary approaches are usually a bit more collaborative in that various professionals might, at least informally, discuss the client and try to cooperate on goals. There are still separate treatment sessions for each discipline, but perhaps the biggest difference between multi- and interdisciplinary cooperation is that there is a bit more joint goal setting and communication among the professionals.

In transdisciplinary collaboration there is the most communication and cooperation among professionals. The psychologist may actually work on communication goals at the same time as behavioral objectives. The SLP might incorporate motor skills into the treatment sessions for communication goals. The classroom teacher might assist in communication goals in the context of the classroom. There is a large literature on consultative models used in assessment and treatment and it is beyond the scope of this text to elaborate on this research (Damico, 1987; Ferguson, 1991; Frassinelli, Superior, & Meyers, 1983; Fujiki & Brinton, 1984; Magnotta, 1991; Marvin, 1987; Montgomery, 1992; Moore-Brown, 1991).

It is important; however, for beginning practicum students to see that, depending on where you are doing therapy, you may experience a variety of types of treatment approaches. Each of these different models of treatment involves changes in the types of professional verbal interactions you will have with other disciplines. These range from very little communication and collaboration (multidisciplinary) to frequent and close communication and collaboration (transdisciplinary). You should be able to see at this point that in multidisciplinary approaches you are pretty much on your own in terms of assessing, developing goals, providing treatment, and evaluating treatment progress. On the other hand, in a transdisciplinary model you will have to communicate and cooperate with all the other disciplines involved to assess, develop goals, provide treatment, and evaluate treatment outcomes. In such a model you might be doing your therapy in the classroom environment instead of a therapy room. You may also be reinforcing academic goals in your therapy and behavioral goals suggested by the psychologist. In transdisciplinary models, everything is negotiated among the professionals involved, and this is all done by means of verbal communication. Some guidelines for conducting collaboration with other professionals were presented by Haynes et al. (2006). We briefly paraphrase some of those points below.

Administrative matters:

- When using a collaborative model, it should not be an informal process, but should be formalized at a meeting. The group of professionals should assemble and discuss the collaborative treatment approach for the client.
- After the discussion, someone on the team should be designated to write down the treatment approach and everyone's responsibilities so that it can be included in the client's folder.

Attitudinal variables:

- You should listen attentively to other professionals on the team and "show respect and consideration for the other team members' expertise, questions, opinions, decisions, concerns, or goals involving the client" (Haynes et al., 2006, p. 33).
- You should assume a positive attitude and be sure to reinforce other professionals for their good ideas.

- Make sure you have studied the client's folder and have some issues/concerns that you want to address to the group.

Conducting meetings:

- Make sure that each professional has an opportunity to provide input.
- Use "situational leadership" in which the professional with the most expertise on an issue (e.g., psychologist, SLP, teacher, PT, OT) takes the lead in discussing the topic.
- It is important for team members not to come to the meeting with a preconceived idea of what will be done. This is not working on a team; it is assuming that you have the best idea and it should be implemented. These meetings are not designed for one person to convince the other professionals to approach the treatment according to a single perspective or plan. The group should discuss the tactics for dealing with the problem and devise a joint approach to accomplishing goals.
- Do not use too much discipline-specific jargon. This interferes with communication and is a subtle way of putting other team members in a subservient position of having to ask for clarification.
- The team should devise specific goals for the client, assign responsibilities for targeting them, and discuss how they will be evaluated and who will assess the progress toward the goals.
- As mentioned above, this should be formalized in a report following the meeting and included in the client's folder.

No doubt, you can see that collaborating with other disciplines takes time, planning, preparation, and professional verbal communication.

Solving Problems in Informal Daily Interactions

In any relationship, including professional ones, there is always the possibility that interpersonal difficulties can arise. Although there are many areas in which interpersonal problems can occur, in our experience there are three major categories likely to be encountered by beginning students in clinical practicum: (a) mistakes, (b) misunderstanding/miscommunication, and (c) crossing discipline boundaries.

Making Mistakes

The first area of interpersonal difficulty involves making errors or mistakes in assessment, treatment, or clinical reporting. First of all, *everyone* makes mistakes at some point. You tend to make fewer mistakes with experience, so students in training are a "high-risk" population. Hopefully, your clinical supervisor can help you head off major errors, but there are always some that slip through. One thing is certain: once you make an error you should learn from that experience and not let it happen again. That is one difference between you and your clinical supervisor: The supervisor has had the opportunity to make errors over a long period of time and learn from those mistakes, and you are only beginning. What kinds of mistakes are we talking about? Obviously, you will make many mistakes in writing clinical reports, but those are between you and your supervisor. Those errors never make it out into the world for others to see. In verbal communication, however, you do not have the luxury of a rough draft and soliciting comments from your supervisor. Thus, those verbal errors are not as easily retrievable. For example, you might have given information at a staffing that was incorrect or misinterpreted. In this case, the other professionals on the team may not know that the scores you presented were wrong and take them at face value. Obviously, if you said the child scored in the 80th percentile on a language test, but it was really the 8th percentile, this represents a major discrepancy. In cases like this, it is important for you to admit your mistake as soon as possible and explain the true nature of the situation. Everyone makes mistakes; it is only when you do not acknowledge them or try to hide them that you get into trouble. Other professionals will respect you more for finding and admitting your error than if you did not report it at all. Imagine your embarrassment, if after working with the client for a long time some other professional finds a discrepancy and brings it to the attention of the group at the next staffing.

The same principle applies to treatment objectives. Let's say you recommended in a staffing that certain goals should be a priority for language intervention. After working with the client for a while, you realize that the goals you set were far too ambitious and difficult for the client and you need to select other goals that are more realistic. Other professionals will respect your clinical decision to change your goals after considering the client's performance.

Because we know that students in training are mistake-prone, there are several proactive principles to keep in mind. First, you should check and double-check your work so that mistakes can be found and corrected before you communicate them verbally. You cannot do a good job of professional verbal communication if you are relying on inaccurate data. A second principle to keep in mind is to think about what you are planning to say before you open your mouth. Make sure it is based on accurate data and not speculation. Make sure you think about saying it as professionally as possible. If you are not sure, ask someone such as a mentor or supervisor who is willing to provide helpful advice. Remember, once you say something, it is out there in the environment. You cannot, as they say, "un-ring a bell."

Misunderstandings and Miscommunications

Another area of potential difficulty with other professionals is misunderstanding and miscommunication. This is not just limited to the use of technical, discipline-specific language; it can come at you from many directions. The box shows some examples.

> **OT:** Mr. Smith's family told me that you said he will not ever be able to feed himself. Feeding is one of our major goals and I don't appreciate you telling the family he won't be able to do it.
>
> (Actually, you only said to the family that Mr. Smith was having some difficulty with feeding himself, among other aspects of activities of daily living, including communication. You never said anything about prognosis or the future. This was a misunderstanding and exaggeration by the family that was passed on to the OT).

Teacher: Bobby's parents told me at our conference last week that you said I wasn't doing a very good job of teaching him how to read. I don't like it when other people undermine what I'm trying to do in the classroom.

(Actually, you said to the parents that children with language impairment often have difficulty learning to read and might need some extra help from time to time. The parents interpreted this as the teacher not doing her job.)

SLP: Johnny seems to be missing many of the cognitive attainments that are associated with language development.

Psychologist: SLPs are not qualified to assess intelligence; that is the job of the psychologist!

(Actually, you were only talking about certain cognitive play behaviors such as object permanence, means-end, symbolic play, and functional use of objects that are related to language development. You were not making judgments about his overall intelligence.)

School Principal: My teachers tell me that you are complaining about the room that you use for speech therapy. You need to know that we have space limitations here and everyone cannot have exactly the type of room they want.

(Actually, you did say to two teachers that, because you were assigned to work in the cafeteria on the stage behind the curtain, it was a bit noisy for some of the distractible students, especially when the custodial and kitchen staff were setting up for lunchtime.)

All of these situations were the product of misinterpretation or miscommunication among various professionals. In each of the instances the result was one professional being upset because of something someone thought you had said or done. These situations are unavoidable due to human nature. People do not always render an accurate report of what others have said, and the result is misunderstanding. If these situations are not dealt with, it could result in damaging the professional relationship you have with people from other disciplines. As a result, it could lead to unsuccessful collaborations and ultimately hurt the clients we are trying to serve.

In all of these situations, the antidote is effective professional verbal communication. First, it is important to notice the fact that a person is upset over something she feels you have done. This may be communicated directly as in the above examples, or indirectly by nonverbal cues or reports from others. Again, it is important to look at both content and affect of what someone says to you. Once you perceive there might be a problem, you need to confront it as soon as possible. Negative feelings incubate and typically grow worse without bringing them out into the open. So you need to communicate to the other person that you understand what she is feeling.

In the first example above, you might say something like, "That kind of statement is very upsetting to me, and I know it must be to you as well. I know that you are working on feeding, and if the family wants to know about prognosis, they need to talk to you. Let me see if I can clarify what happened. The family was expressing some frustration about how little progress he was making. I recall telling the family that Mr. Smith had difficulty in many areas including communication, movement, feeding, and cognitive issues and that it is a challenge to have so many things to work on at the same time. I don't know how they translated that into a negative prognosis for feeding, but I'm sorry for the misunderstanding. I would never make statements to a family about something in your field. You are the expert on those issues, and I value our working relationship." Notice several things. First, the response validates the person's feelings about being upset. Second, the response tries to address the concern directly and put it in the context of what actually occurred. Finally, the tone of the response gave respect to the other professional's expertise and role in dealing with feeding issues. It might have been easy for the OT to just ignore the comments from the family, but if that happened, resentment could build for the SLP and a relationship could be impaired. It is always good to confront such issues head on. If there is a logical explanation or misunderstanding, most people will accept this as a resolution to their concern. If, on the other hand, you have made a mistake or a misstatement or have actually said an unprofessional remark, you need to apologize for it and move on. It is easy to misspeak or to make a statement in confidence to someone you trust, only to have it revealed at a later time. Optimally, it is a good policy to never say anything that you do not want another person to hear.

A final area of possible communication difficulty with other professionals revolves around crossing discipline boundaries. Professionals are known to exhibit a certain amount of "turfism," meaning that they perceive specific areas and procedures to be part of their field and no other's. If another professional "steps on their turf" they become defensive and upset. Because communication sciences and disorders overlap with many other disciplines, it is not unusual for us to inadvertently step over a line or two as we deal with other professionals. Think about it. We deal with teachers, nurses, physicians, psychologists, administrators, OTs, PTs, social workers, and other SLPs. Many of the issues we confront are the same as those dealt with by other professions. Take behavior problems as an example. Any professional that deals with a child who exhibits behavior disturbances must deal with these issues at the same time she is trying to accomplish the goals in her field of expertise. Thus, the teacher must deal with behavior during the teaching of science. The psychologist must deal with behaviors while teaching the student how to cope with them. The SLP deals with behaviors while teaching language and pragmatics to the student. At a staffing, it would be easy for the SLP to describe "the best way" to deal with behavior problems, but you can see that this risks stepping on the boundaries of the psychologist. Diplomacy is very important in professional verbal communication. It is better to say, "I'm not the authority on how to best deal with these behaviors, but here is what I have been doing in language therapy. I would be interested to get some input from Mr. Jones (psychologist) on this issue." In this example, you admit that behavior problems must be dealt with in your treatment sessions, but you also defer to the psychologist in terms of soliciting suggestions from the person who may be more qualified in behavior disturbance. In many work settings, disturbances in professional relationships can often be traced back to one person stepping on another's turf. Be wary of this next time you are tempted to give advice on topics that are only ancillary to your area of expertise.

This chapter focused on professional verbal communication with people from other disciplines. There are many pitfalls in professional relationships, and although verbal communication is often the cause of interpersonal difficulties, it is also the solution. Keep the channels of communication open, and you will be on your way to becoming a competent and qualified professional.

11 Interacting with Individuals from Diverse Backgrounds

INTRODUCTION

It is estimated that one in every 10 Americans, across all ages, races, and genders, has experienced or lived with some type of communication disorder (including speech, language and hearing disorders), and that nearly 6 million children under the age of 18 have a speech or language disorder (NIDCD, 2009). With an estimated 312.7 million people in the United States (U.S. Census Bureau, Population Estimates, 2012), this encompasses an incredibly large group of people. Interestingly, the U.S. Census also shows that the number of foreign-born residents is projected to rise from 31 million in 2000 to 48 million in 2025. The Hispanic population alone (the largest minority group) is projected to triple by mid-century, and Asian Pacific Americans, the fastest growing ethnic group, includes more than 60 separate groups. In addition, the latest Census data indicate that almost 14% of U.S. residents do not speak English, creating a challenging clinical environment for speech-language pathologists and audiologists.

Across most service-related disciplines, the issue of multicultural diversity is a much publicized, and much criticized topic. Much publicized, because of the significant demographic changes that are taking place in the United States, and much criticized because clinical educators and students agree that most health professional programs fall short in preparing students to work with culturally diverse individuals. And in the field of speech-language pathology, this is no exception. In an article on its website, The American Speech-Language-Hearing Association (ASHA) addressed the issue directly. According to the article, "ASHA has targeted increasing the cultural competence of speech-language pathologists (SLPs) and audiologists as a strategic objective in its pathway to excellence" (2008). As a result, there have been a number of initiatives on the part of ASHA to promote cultural diversity. This is mostly due to clinicians and educators continuing to report concerns regarding the provision of services to culturally and linguistically diverse individuals.

CULTURAL COMPETENCE AND THE SLP

What is cultural competence? In short, it is developing an awareness and understanding of how individuals interact in the world based on the philosophy and beliefs of the culture to which they belong. Students in speech-language pathology will have numerous opportunities to meet and form relationships with people from a myriad of backgrounds and across the life span. Becoming culturally competent will ensure that you are well prepared to assist any person with a communication disorder, regardless of their background, or to what degree it is similar or different from yours. There has been a great deal of research on multicultural issues, and how they affect the client/clinician relationship. Suffice it to say that we do not cover the depth and breadth of that information in this chapter. What we hope to do, however, is to give you an idea of how you can begin to start moving toward cross-cultural competence, even as a beginning clinician.

Stewart and Gonzalez (2002), in an article on the role of SLP graduate programs in preparing student clinicians to serve a diverse population identified multicultural training goals for SLPs that include: increasing diversity of SLPs, increasing the quantity and quality of research, and improving academic and clinical preparation. It is to this end that we felt it necessary to introduce the speech-language pathology student to multicultural issues regarding their clinical practicum experience in order to facilitate their growth into a competent clinician.

There is no question that students in the field of speech-language pathology will be faced with understanding how to interact with and quite possibly counsel individuals from diverse backgrounds. One way to improve your skills as a clinician is to develop cultural sensitivity, or a willingness to learn about and address the needs of *every* patient. Working with someone from a culture that differs from yours naturally creates an opportunity for you to establish rapport and communicate effectively with this person, simply due to the fact that you are aware of their cultural differences. As a result, you are probably more sensitive to cultural norms and mores, and take great care in making sure you honor those. Most people are keenly aware when someone looks, talks, or acts differently than people from their own culture and background. You may even become aware that "your way" of communicating with someone may not be appropriate, effective or even understood. It is always important to put yourself in someone else's shoes, as the saying goes, in order to truly establish a positive, successful relationship. As stated by Battle (2002), when counseling individuals from diverse cultural backgrounds, it is important to adhere to a basic set of guidelines, which can be best explained as a three-step process:

1. Counseling should begin during the initial evaluation so that the client and their family members or caregivers understand what will take place. The clinician will want to be aware of cultural beliefs about the necessity of the intervention process.
2. The clinician should always make sure the client and/or family members understand the diagnosis, prognosis and any therapy techniques that may not be straightforward. Clinicians should remember to observe rules for cultural interaction (verbal, nonverbal, and social).
3. The clinician should be aware of personal adjustments of the clients and significant others as an ongoing part of the treatment process. It is

important that the clinician explore the possible significance of cultural mores and rules with regard to cultural identity and/or generational factors (age and maturity).

Even though a clinician may have a desire and a willingness to learn about others, it is impossible to learn everything about different cultures. Table 11–1 is a guide to various social interaction styles of the largest minority groups living in the United States in comparison to Anglo-European or American culture. It is our hope that this information will be beneficial to the SLP in following the guidelines mentioned above.

According to ASHA, "Culture can be viewed broadly as the socially constructed and learned ways of believing that identify groups of people, and verbal, as well as nonverbal communication behaviors readily identify cultural groups" (2004). Additionally, culture has been more specifically defined as integrated patterns of human behavior that include the language, thoughts, customs, beliefs, values and institutions of racial, ethnic, religious, or social groups. Cultural competence is the development of a set of behaviors, attitudes and policies that come together in a system, agency or among professionals that enables effective work in cross-cultural situations. According to the Office of Minority Health, a division of the U.S. Department of Health and Human Services, "cultural competence is important because health care services that are respectful of and responsive to the health beliefs, practices and cultural and linguistic needs of diverse patients can help bring about positive health outcomes."

Let's examine how cultural competence ties in with delivery of speech-language pathology services, whether in the university clinic, public schools or medical settings. When the SLP enters into a clinical or therapeutic relationship with clients and their families, caregivers or significant others, there may be some preconceived ideas about the individual. This could be based on the patient's name, age, referral source, place of birth, or even their diagnosis. It is natural for people to make assumptions about someone they have never met based on certain factors. Unfortunately, these assumptions are often prejudiced, discriminatory or simply inaccurate. A good clinician doesn't allow stereotypes, judgments, or

Table 11–1. Greeting and Customs for Interacting Among Various Racial and Ethnic Groups

Ethnic or Racial Group	Greetings	Customs for Interaction or Visiting
Anglo-European American	• Warm, firm handshakes with direct eye contact is expected • An arm's length is considered one's personal space that should not be violated • Males usually shake hands with males, although there are no rules against women shaking hands with men or young persons shaking hands with the elderly • Turn-taking during conversation is important • Personal topics, personal self-disclosure, and controversial issues are avoided	• Punctuality is expected • Direct, face-to-face communication is expected • Personal opinions are expressed openly
African-American	• Address by surnames and title (e.g., Mr., Mrs., Miss, etc.) unless permission is granted to use first names	• Avoid telling the family that they are touchy about racial issues • Avoid racial jokes even about one's own culture • Avoid stereotyping African American families • Don't talk with coworkers about personal matters • Don't judge family function by socioeconomic status
Asian-American	• Address by surname • Avoid prolonged eye contact • Avoid physical touching • Greet family members from oldest to youngest Handshaking • Only males shake hands • Youngsters do not shake hands with elders	• Avoid personal questions during initial contact • Remove shoes when entering the home • Sit with feet flat on the floor and hands folded in your lap • Accept food or drink if offered • Demonstrate emotional restraint
Latin American	• Speak to husband before the wife if both are present • Use a calm tone of voice • Initial "small talk" is important for establishing rapport • Provide background about what can be expected in future interactions	• Respect cultural artifacts/rituals and their importance to the family • Don't rush or be impatient, which shows disrespect • Don't be too direct • Build interpersonal relationships • Sit with good posture • Avoid the term "illegal alien"; use the term "undocumented immigrant" instead

continues

Table 11–1. *continued*

Ethnic or Racial Group	Greetings	Customs for Interaction or Visiting
Middle-Eastern American	• Personal space or social distance is shorter than for Anglo-European Americans • Men may kiss other men on the cheek upon greeting • Women may exchange hugs and/or kisses upon greeting • Avoid direct or assertive communication	• Remove shoes when entering the home unless family does not • Accept food and/or drink if offered and partake in the hospitality • Do not sit with your back to an adult who is present • Sit with legs up or crossed in front • Stand when new guests arrive, particularly the elderly
Native American	• Initial "small talk" is important for establishing rapport • Provide background about what can be expected in future interaction	• May not answer knocks at the door or doorbell • Ask whether an appointment is convenient (scheduling a time many not be as good) • Ask family where they would like you to sit • Family members may come and go from the home • Confidential topics may best be handled in the office • Accept food and/or drink and partake in the hospitality. • In rural areas, unscheduled visits should be signaled by a honking of a car horn

Source: Based on *Developing Cross-Cultural Competence: A Guide for Working with Children and Their Families* (2nd edition), by E. W. Lynch and M. J. Hanson, 1997, Baltimore, MD: Brookes.

preconceived notions to affect their ability to thoroughly assess and outline an effective treatment plan for clients who may be from a different culture than their own. A good clinician looks at the therapeutic relationship as one that both parties (the client and the SLP) can learn, and optimally benefit from.

THE THERAPEUTIC CYCLE

According to Johnson (2012), it is important for clinicians to realize that various aspects of culture such as customs, learning styles, beliefs/values, and social interaction style may influence the cycle of activities in a therapeutic relationship. The cycle of activi-

ties, or the cycle of the therapeutic relationship, as described by Stockman, Boult, and Robinson (2004), is defined as follows:

- Referring: providing access to clinical services
- Scheduling: selecting the time for a patient to receive clinical services
- Gathering information: obtaining patients' pertinent background information
- Assessing: determining the nature of a patient's communication disorder
- Recommending: advising and/or counseling the patient about potential treatment plans
- Treating: ameliorating or lessening the impact of the patient's communication disorder
- Discharging: terminating the therapeutic relationship

In this section, we examine each aspect of the cycle in a little more detail.

1. *Referring:* Even with specific programs in place such as Child Find, Early Intervention, Medicaid screenings, and well-baby visits to pediatricians, cultural and linguistic barriers often prevent young children from getting the help they need. Parents who do not speak English may not understand the purpose of the screenings, the importance of follow-up testing or the need for referrals to other professionals. This is where an interpreter can make the difference in a child or an adult receiving the intervention necessary to improve their quality of life.

2. *Scheduling:* A referral usually results in scheduling an appointment with a speech-language pathologist, whether at a private clinic, public school, or university clinic. Again, parents from culturally diverse backgrounds may not follow through if they don't know the reason for the appointment. They may also be apprehensive about returning calls to unfamiliar, English-speaking individuals. According to Johnson (2012), "Families of culturally and linguistically diverse backgrounds may value punctuality differently than mainstream culture and may be late to their scheduled appointments. Western cultures value punctuality more than Latino, Native American and African American cultures do (p. 57)." She also adds that clinicians should exercise positive regard and consider that tardiness to appointments may be due to cultural differences rather than a lack of respect.

3. *Gathering Information:* Obtaining information for the patient's case history may be difficult, especially if the patient or caregiver does not speak English well. Having an interpreter to assist in filling out this form, or even having a form written in Spanish or another language would be beneficial. Be advised, however, that individuals from some cultures are reluctant to share personal information with professionals; therefore, this may also be a barrier to obtaining an accurate case history.

4. *Assessing:* This may be difficult for a myriad of reasons; some of which are quite obvious. Patients (children or adults) will not be able to respond appropriately to an assessment tool if they do not know what to do. In this situation, use of an interpreter is highly recommended. If an interpreter is not available, family members may be able to assist with communication. In some clinics, Spanish versions of commonly used speech and language assessments are available. The speech-language pathologist uses every resource possible to obtain valid assessment results.

5. *Recommending, Advising, and Counseling:* this includes advising and counseling patients and families about the diagnostic results and possible treatment plans. The impact of a particular diagnosis for a child or adult with a communication disorder can be difficult for parents or caregivers to hear. For families who do not speak English, it is advisable to utilize an interpreter, or a professional who speaks their language. This is where informational counseling comes into play. The ability to tolerate "clinical silence" has been emphasized throughout the literature. In this country, most people feel uncomfortable with silence during conversations. It is often interpreted as negative or indicating tension. In contrast, for individuals in other ethnic or cultural groups (Asian, Native American, Middle Eastern), silence is seen as appropriate and positive (Battle, 1997). Therefore, one of the most powerful techniques for maintaining a client-centered focus is for the SLP to permit and tolerate silence during the interview (Capuzzi & Gross, 2003). Refer back to the guidelines in Chapter 9 regarding this type of counseling.

6. *Treating:* Explanations of possible treatment options should, if at all possible, be in the patient's native language, whether through a bilingual SLP, or an interpreter. It is advantageous to provide non-English-speaking patients or caregivers with written information in their native language describing as many details as possible regarding the treatment plan. Also, once the treatment begins, the SLP should be aware of cultural differences regarding communication styles.

7. *Discharging:* When terminating the therapeutic relationship, the SLP may provide the patient, caregivers or parents with recommendations for

a home program or other follow-up. This, again, should be explained through an interpreter, or someone who speaks the patient's native language. If other recommendations are made, the SLP should be aware that the family of the patient may not follow through due to cultural differences.

Whether in the university clinic, the public schools or a medical setting, graduate students in speech-language pathology will be introduced to and gain experience in all of the components of the "cycle of activities." Some health care professions require more cross-cultural competence than others. Specialists in communication sciences and disorders require a greater degree of cross-cultural competence than some other professionals, who see patients for one visit with little need for extensive follow-up. Speech-language pathologists, however, assess and remediate patients' communication abilities, which are deeply rooted in their native cultures (Johnson, 2012).

In closing, we felt it was important to include ASHA's position statement regarding cultural competence as stated in Horton-Ikard and Munoz (2010). This document was developed to provide guidance to ASHA members and certificate holders as they provide ethically appropriate services to all populations, while recognizing their own cultural/linguistic background, and that of their clients or patients.

- Certain materials may be inappropriate and even offensive to some individuals.
- Families may choose complementary and alternative medicine, traditional healing practices, and different communication styles, as opposed to mainstream diagnostic and therapeutic approaches. The clinician must have the cultural competence to accommodate these needs and choices, or at a minimum know when and where to seek assistance.
- The clinician must be aware that "differences" do not imply "deficiencies."

- When a clinician is not proficient in the language used by the client and family, a suitable interpreter should be used. The use of interpreters and others who are proficient in the language of the client and family does not negate the ultimate responsibility of the clinician in diagnosing and/or treating the client/patient.
- A clinician must remember that bilingual skill (understanding and speaking the language) does not equate to bicultural skill (understanding and respecting the culture)—both are necessary for culturally competent service delivery.
- Beliefs and values unique to the individual clinician-client encounter must be understood, protected and respected. Care must be taken not to make assumptions about individuals based upon their particular culture, ethnicity, language, or life experiences that could lead to misdiagnosis or improper treatment of the client/patient.
- Providers must enter into the relationship with awareness, knowledge, and skills about their own culture and cultural biases.
- To address the unique, individual characteristics and cultural background of clients and their families, providers should be prepared to be open and flexible in the selection, administration and interpretation of diagnostic and/or treatment regimens.
- When cultural or linguistic differences may negatively influence outcomes, referral to or collaboration with others with needed knowledge, skills and/or experience is indicated.

In summary, speech-language pathologists must develop cross-cultural competence in order to provide relevant interventions for patients and their families as part of serving a diverse population across the life span. Becoming competent in our profession demands that we are not only knowledgeable of racial, ethnic, and/or linguistic differences and their effects on service delivery, but also responsive to the needs of our diverse patient population.

12 Interacting with Supervisors

Communication takes many forms in our field including written, electronic, group discussion, and individual conversation. The importance of one-on-one conversation in our field cannot be overemphasized. We do it with colleagues, supervisors, clients, other professionals, parents, and family members. Part of professional communication is learning how to address these various constituencies in conversational interactions. In some cases we have these conversations just as a social interchange. At other times, the conversation has a distinct goal such as persuasion, motivation, justification, or counseling. In the previous three chapters we discussed professional verbal communication with clients/families, individuals from diverse backgrounds, and with professionals from other disciplines. We addressed some of the problems that arise and how professional verbal communication can be used to resolve them. This chapter deals with verbal communication that takes place between supervisors and student clinicians. As you will learn during your training, the first clinical supervisors you will encounter are in the university speech and hearing clinic. As you progress in your program you will no doubt be sent off campus to schools, hospitals, rehabilitation centers, community clinics, private practices, and long-term care facilities. In each of these work settings you will be under the direction of a clinical supervisor. As mentioned in Chapter 2, there are distinct differences between the university clinic and these other settings. The communication issues and student mistakes mentioned in this chapter can occur in any practicum setting, so we remind students to be proactive and maintain an open line of professional communication with your supervisors. Although the information generally applies to all practicum settings, we want to remind you that once you leave the university clinic, everything moves faster. You will be seeing more clients, the schedule will be more hectic, the paperwork deadlines are shorter, and there is less tolerance for practicum student mistakes. These differences are, in large part, due to the fact that you are now working in a facility or school system where professional service delivery is expected and demanded. In the university clinic, everyone knows that it is a training program and the therapy is conducted by students under supervision. In a hospital, school, or rehabilitation facility, most of the service providers are certified professionals and students are in the minority. Also, your supervisor will not have 20 different practicum students on whom to focus. Therefore, it is possible that you will receive increased supervisory attention as compared to your experiences at the university clinic.

Interestingly, practicum students often report two different scenarios in off-campus settings. The first situation involves a more intensive supervisor-student relationship. This is the product of (a) more clients seen by the same student and supervisor and (b) fewer students to deal with on the part of the supervisor. The result is more time together talking about cases. Because the supervisor only has one or two students to supervise, more time can be spent scrutinizing your behavior. The second scenario reported by students at off-campus sites is less time available for supervisory conferencing. Because the supervisor is busy seeing clients and going to meetings, there is less time for supervisory conferences and, thus, less direction for the student. Some students liken this to being thrown into a swimming pool and told, "Now, learn to swim!" They report less time for the supervisor to explain and model techniques and elaborate on the required paperwork.

Either of the above scenarios can be disconcerting to a practicum student, but take our word for it, the student does learn in either one. In off-campus clinical environments you will no doubt feel more stress than you did in the sheltered environment of the university clinic, and this stress leads to unique problems between supervisors and students. But we are getting ahead of our story. First, we talk about the nature of the relationship between a practicum student and a clinical supervisor.

THE EVOLUTION OF STUDENT AND SUPERVISOR RELATIONSHIP THROUGH THE PRACTICUM EXPERIENCE

Whether you know it or not, training programs are designed in such a way as to generate particular expectations on the part of students and supervisors. These expectations change in a predictable way as the student progresses through practicum. Anderson (1988) suggested a continuum of supervision showing that supervision is adapted to the situation and needs of the supervisee. As participation by the student increases, the degree of involvement by the supervisor decreases. The aim, of course, is to develop independent clinicians who are capable of self-supervision. Our own version of this relationship is shown in Figure 12–1, which depicts this change as the lesson of the linking triangles. The triangle on the left with the dotted outline represents the clinical supervisor. The triangle on the right with the solid line represents the student. The height of each triangle represents the amount of clinical responsibility allocated to supervisor and student as time progresses in the training program. So you can see that the supervisor has a lot of clinical responsibility at the beginning of your undergraduate program as indicated by the height of the arrow indicating clinical responsibility. Note that as time goes on, the supervisor's triangle starts to narrow in terms of clinical responsibility. At the end of your graduate program, the supervisor's triangle has come to a point and indicates almost no clinical responsibility. Now look at the student triangle. The student starts the training program with very little clinical responsibility as shown by the pointed end of the triangle.

As the students make their way through the program, the student triangle begins to broaden until at the end of graduate school the student is taking most of the clinical responsibility. The triangles of the supervisor and student are exactly opposite of one another as time goes by.

This phenomenon of student practicum experience suggests that you change as you progress through your training. As a beginning student you know little practical application of your classroom materials, and with experience you become more adept at planning, executing, and reporting clinical activities. This is a natural progression for students as they become more professional and competent. The lesson here is that you should not expect to be the same in your clinical abilities at the end of your graduate program as you were as a beginning practicum student. The transformation of a student from novice to competent clinician also holds a lesson for clinical supervisors. It is axiomatic that supervisors have a sliding scale of expectations when dealing with students in training. For instance, a supervisor has much lower expectations of a beginning undergraduate student as compared to a last semester graduate student. It is only logical that expectations and grading criteria change over time in a training program. Thus, if you continue to behave as a beginning undergraduate student in terms of taking clinical responsibility, your clinical practicum grade will suffer as time goes by. The expectation is that you will profit from your classroom work and practicum experiences to become more self-reliant and take more clinical responsibility for your cases.

Sometimes a source of difficulty between students and supervisors is a mismatch of expectations between the two individuals. For example, your supervisor may be expecting you to take more clinical responsibility as you approach your third semester in practicum, and you might still feel the need for more help and direction by your supervisor. This mismatch can result in frustration for both parties and a lower grade in practicum for the student. Remember, during your clinical evolution the expectations of supervisors steadily increase based on your past practicum experience. You will know when such a mismatch in expectations occurs when supervisors ask you to independently plan, ask you for rationales, and ask you to research your classroom notes for hints

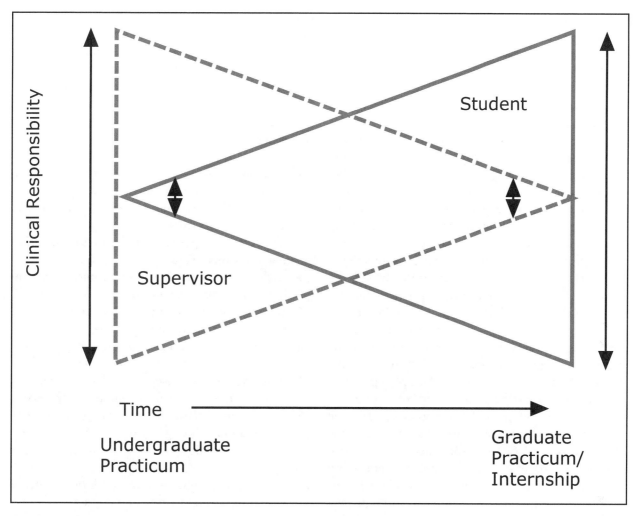

Figure 12–1. How clinical responsibility changes over time in a training program.

on how to handle your client. Another symptom of the mismatch is when a supervisor laments having to "spoon-feed" you as a practicum student. This is your cue to actively take more clinical responsibility and come to planning sessions with your own ideas instead of waiting to be directed by your supervisor.

THE SUPERVISORY RELATIONSHIP

The relationship between the practicum student, clinical supervisor, and client is a unique blend of service delivery, clinical teaching, and student learning. Although the major goal must be the clinical

progress and welfare of the client, this is also used as a teaching-learning experience between supervisor and student. In an ideal relationship, the client makes optimal progress, the supervisor can accomplish teaching goals for the student, and the student learns the targeted clinical skills. Sometimes it works exactly this way, but other times there is an imbalance. You can well imagine that this is a very difficult balancing act. The supervisor is not simply doing therapy by proxy using the student as a delivery system. The student is not a neutral conduit through which the supervisor dispenses treatment to the client. True, the student delivers the therapy and learns the critical skills of listening, motivating, taking data, and interpersonal communication abilities with clients.

But the student training goal goes beyond the face-to-face skills that occur in the treatment room. In supervisory conferences, the practicum student must learn to understand *why* the treatment goals were selected, how they were arranged in the appropriate sequence, and the proper way to conduct tasks with the client.

Even after all of this preparation, an unavoidable part of clinical practicum is that the student will still make errors in judgment and behavior. Making mistakes and problem solving how to correct them is a valuable part of the learning process. If the goal of a university clinic or practicum setting was simply to do the best therapy for the client, the supervisor would provide the treatment. Clearly, in a practicum experience, there are treatment goals that benefit the client and teaching-learning goals that benefit the student. Obviously, student mistakes can have a negative effect on client progress, so the supervisor must do something to compensate for this. In most cases, the supervisor helps to ensure that the student attacks the client's problem with the very best plan possible. Supervisors do not have the luxury of letting students come up with plans that are not optimal for the client merely to further the cause of student learning. Thus, the supervisor helps the student to generate a sound therapeutic procedure and to understand how and why that procedure was developed. This is done in a supervisory conference through professional verbal communication. Another way that the supervisor "levels the playing field" for the client is to physically supervise many of the treatment sessions or demonstrate specific therapy techniques to make sure the student is carrying out the plan optimally. Typically, less experienced students are supervised more intensively than more experienced students. Although ASHA demands that sessions are supervised a minimum of 25% of the time, most supervisors provide as much oversight as needed, depending on the capabilities of the student and the complexity of the client's disorder.

Goals of Supervisors and Students

The ASHA Committee on Supervision (1985) outlined a number of tasks that supervisors might be expected to perform during practicum experiences with stu-

dents. Hegde and Davis (2010) explain each of these tasks in more detail, and students are referred to this source for a more descriptive summary. We only list the tasks expected to be performed by supervisors and students to provide you with an overview. Most of the tasks are relatively self-explanatory. First, we can expect clinical supervisors to perform the following:

1. Establishing and maintaining an effective working relationship with the supervisee
2. Assisting the supervisee in developing clinical goals and objectives
3. Assisting the supervisee in developing and refining assessment skills
4. Assisting the supervisee in developing and refining clinical management skills
5. Demonstrating for and participating with the supervisee in the clinical process
6. Assisting the supervisee in observing and analyzing assessment and treatment sessions
7. Assisting the supervisee in the development and maintenance of clinical and supervisory records
8. Interacting with the supervisee in planning, executing and analyzing supervisory conferences
9. Assisting the supervisee in evaluation of clinical performance
10. Assisting the supervisee in developing skills of verbal reporting, writing and editing
11. Sharing information regarding ethical, legal, regulatory and reimbursement aspects of the profession
12. Modeling and facilitating professional conduct
13. Demonstrating research skills in the clinical or supervisor process

Similarly, Hegde and Davis (2010) discuss a number of expectations that a supervisor might have of practicum students. Practicum students should demonstrate the following:

■ Compliance with the Code of Ethics of the American Speech-Language-Hearing Association.
■ Knowledge of ASHA's preferred practice patterns and scope of practice.
■ Knowledge of and conformity to the clinic's policies and procedures.
■ Ensuring client confidentiality.

▓ Appreciating the cultural and personal background of the client.

▓ Evidence planning and preparation for every treatment or assessment session.

▓ Knowledge of appropriate diagnostic and treatment methods in terms of test instruments and therapy approaches.

▓ Demonstration of an ability to develop appropriate goals for assessment and treatment sessions.

▓ Demonstration of the ability to be punctual with both written assignments and supervisory conferences.

▓ Maintaining accurate and appropriate clinical records.

▓ Showing the ability to apply coursework information to the client and engaging in appropriate library research when existing information is not available from classes.

▓ Demonstrating the ability to ask appropriate questions of the supervisor in order to use this mentor as a clinical resource.

▓ Exhibiting the ability to engage in self-evaluation of clinical skills

▓ Demonstration of punctual and regular attendance to assessment/treatment sessions.

▓ Showing the ability to accurately maintain records of clinical clock hours and information for certification forms such as Knowledge and Skill Assessment (KASA) documents.

▓ Demonstration of the ability to act, talk, and write in a professional manner.

▓ Maintaining open lines of communication with the clinical supervisor and reporting any concerns or significant events in a timely manner.

It is easy to see that the goals of supervisors and students overlap significantly. For instance, the supervisor wants to show the student how to develop effective assessment/treatment strategies, and this is one of the student's goals as well. From reading the above bullet points you can see that the relationship between supervisor and practicum student is no mystery. We are well aware of the supervisory goals and the learning objectives of the student. However, sometimes putting the teaching and learning goals together creates some difficulties.

CRITICAL DIFFERENCES BETWEEN STUDENTS AND SUPERVISORS

Clinical supervisors and practicum students typically differ in at least three important ways. Some of these differences can cause misperceptions or miscommunications and make the accomplishment of the above-mentioned supervisor and student goals more difficult. Let us compare the clinical supervisor and practicum student:

1. **Credentials, Experience, and Perspective:** The supervisor is usually older than most practicum students and may represent the world view of a more mature individual. Additionally, with age comes attainment of advanced degrees, certification, and licensure. Being a bit older than the student also has allowed for the accumulation of years of clinical and supervision experience. Clearly, the supervisor is "coming from" quite a different perspective than a beginning practicum student, just based on age, training, and experience. In the case of the student, he has little professional experience and fewer degrees and has only begun to embark on career training. There is a large gulf between these individuals that can be difficult to span without mutual respect and effort and professional verbal communication.

2. **Workload:** The supervisor in the university setting is responsible for a caseload of perhaps 20 to 30 clients, and this probably means 20 different students to supervise. Each of these students has a different level of classroom training and clinical experience, so each supervisory conference must be "recalibrated" to account for these variables. An early undergraduate clinician, on the other hand, may have only one or two cases to focus upon. Think of the difference between the supervisor and student just in terms of the caseload size with its attendant differences in clients, student capabilities, different personalities, disparate goals, and varying schedules. It is no wonder that supervisors have a hectic schedule as they move between observation rooms to supervisory conferences to doing paperwork. In many cases these clinical faculty manage to find time to do research and professional projects as

well. It is probably true that the clinical supervisor has a much more complicated schedule than the student even when you count the student's class time.

3. **Teacher-Student Relationship:** Sometimes students beginning practicum forget that the clinical supervisor is as much a teacher as a professor who stands in front of a classroom. There are some practical differences that reinforce this misconception. First, clinical supervision is usually done on an individual teacher-student basis and there is no classroom full of students. Second, we usually meet one-on-one in an office instead of a classroom. Third, because of these individual meetings between supervisor and student there is more of an opportunity to get to know each other as people, unlike the anonymity of the classroom. We raise these differences because they often lead to misconceptions on the part of students beginning the practicum experience. The first misconception is that the practicum does not involve the relationship between a student and a teacher. However, the practicum relationship *is* a teaching-learning experience just like the classroom, except it is highly individualized and very intensive. In a supervisory conference, there is no way to avoid answering a question like you can in the classroom. There is no way to disguise the fact that you are unprepared. Because you cannot hide, you might feel that you can get by on your personal magnetism and scintillating personality. Some students and supervisors may not want to acknowledge the real nature of this relationship and thus cultivate a "friendly" style of interacting. But, no matter how friendly you become with your clinical supervisor, the relationship is always one between a teacher and a student.

Unfortunately, there is always a somewhat adversarial component to a relationship in which one person is in a position to evaluate the performance of another and assign a grade at the end of the semester. The supervisor has the goal of teaching clinical and professional skills, and you the student should have the objective of learning them. Ultimately, the supervisor will have to make judgments about your clinical abilities, professionalism, and how you are progressing toward independence in your practicum experiences. These judgments must be made no matter how cordial the relationship between supervisor and student. Thus, it is a good policy to make your interactions as pleasant and friendly as possible, but at the same time, you must make meaningful and professional contributions to the teaching-learning relationship. Another common mistake made by students is that they sometimes think that there is no homework involved in clinical practicum because it is not a class per se. Again, this idea is a misconception that could lead the student to lower grades and a less than optimal learning experience. Practicum students are expected to "bring something to the table" from their coursework and prior clinical experiences. The supervisor will expect you to go back to your class notes and look up information relevant to your case. Sometimes you will be expected to read articles and book chapters to prepare for clinical work. Obviously, there is a lot of outside work involved in devising clinical materials, keeping track of client data, and writing goals and objectives.

The three areas discussed above can lead to miscommunication on the part of both supervisors and students. Professional verbal communication is necessary to resolve these difficulties.

REMEMBER THE PRINCIPLES OF PROFESSIONAL VERBAL COMMUNICATION

As in professional verbal communication with clients, families, and other professionals, it is important to remember the critical variables of showing respect, being organized, using professional terms, listening and understanding, and paying attention to communicative context. All of these attributes are crucial in dealing with your supervisors. You obviously want to show *respect* for your clinical supervisor because he is experienced, certified, licensed, and in the position of providing you with feedback as well as a grade. *Organization* is important when dealing with supervisors. Typically, there is only a limited amount of time available for a supervisory conference. You should prepare for these conferences just as you prepare for classes or treatment sessions.

For example, you might have specific questions for your supervisor and these should be organized in a logical manner. You should also make sure that the questions you ask cannot be answered by examining your class notes or querying some other source. Your supervisor will be using *professional terminology* in conferences and you should be prepared to do the same. Finally, you must *attend to the communicative context.* When you have a conversation with your supervisor you should attend to content and affect, just as we suggested in communicating with clients or other professionals. Your supervisor might communicate frustration by using intonation, body language, or facial expression rather than words. For instance, your supervisor might say, "Didn't you cover this information in your articulation disorders class?" This could mean that the supervisor wishes you had read your class notes on a particular treatment approach so it would not have to be explained to you in a conference. One of the present authors remembers a student who had a very behaviorally oriented supervisor. The story goes that the student arrived for a supervisory conference without her treatment data from the previous week. The student said, "Oops, I forgot my data." The supervisor replied, "Well, without the treatment data we do not have much to discuss except our opinions, do we? So this conference is over." What is the supervisor's message here? Just the literal translation of the supervisor's words that the conference was terminated? Hardly. The unspoken message was clearly received. That clinician reportedly never came to another supervisory conference without her data for the next 2 years, no matter who was supervising. Do not forget the critical components of professional verbal communication.

COMMUNICATION ISSUES YOU MAY OR MAY NOT ENCOUNTER

When we ask our students about the things that "stress them out" while taking practicum, there is a cluster of complaints that are recycled semester after semester. Interestingly, communication or miscommunication is at the root of most complaints; and all of these issues can be resolved, or at least made more palatable, by acting professionally and using professional verbal communication. Here are some of the most common issues:

1. **Your supervisor wants you to do things that were not addressed in your coursework:** All students enrolled in practicum experiences will develop a relationship with a clinical supervisor. In most cases, this relationship will be a positive one; however, there may be a mismatch between information learned in academic coursework and the goals/activities that the supervisor recommends. Such a mismatch is guaranteed to make the student feel vulnerable, incompetent, and under stress. For instance, the supervisor might recommend assessment or treatment activities that go beyond what was covered in the academic coursework, and the student has to do extra work to learn about this new approach. An example might be that the clinical faculty member has gone to a recent workshop and learned about a technique that applies to the case that you have been assigned. In this scenario you must read articles and handouts that may not be familiar to you from your academic coursework. One way to look at this is that you have been given a chance to learn about a new technique and try to reconcile it with your existing knowledge. Although the extra effort might cause stress in the short term, it is a great opportunity to learn a new treatment approach and actually try it out on a real case.

2. **Your supervisor does not allow you to do things that you learned in coursework:** Academic faculty members will sometimes report that students complain that their supervisor will not let them use techniques or approaches learned in coursework. In most cases, this is due to lack of communication between the academic and clinical faculty, and not a supervisor forbidding the use of a particular approach. When the complaining student is queried, "Did you ask your supervisor if you could add phonological awareness goals to the therapy?" the student most often replies in the negative. Most supervisors would be elated if a student suggested an addition to the treatment regimen that was based on research covered in the classroom. Thus, in most cases it is not the supervisor's fault, but the

timidity of the student in suggesting additions to the treatment plan. There is nothing wrong with asking to use a technique or strategy with your client you learned in the classroom. If it is appropriate, the supervisor will probably go along with it, and if it is not appropriate it provides an opportunity for discussion as to why it should not be used with this particular client. Either way, it is a good learning experience. But you will never know without communicating your concern to your supervisor.

3. **You only have your undergraduate training and are assigned a complicated case:** In most instances, this probably will not happen. Very complicated cases should not be given to a beginning student who has not had the coursework to back up clinical planning. If, however, you are given a complex case, you should expect that supervision will be more intensive. Remember, we said earlier that the main goal of clinical practicum is that the client make progress and not be placed at a disadvantage. No one wants this to happen. If you have a challenging case, be sure to do your part in terms of asking a lot of questions, requesting frequent feedback, and researching issues yourself in addition to the information provided by your supervisor. Again, you must speak up and tell the supervisor that you do not yet feel comfortable with planning the treatment for such a difficult case because you have never had the opportunity before. On the other hand, if you are a graduate student who has worked with many such cases in the past, you have to remember the intersecting triangles in Figure 12–1. In other words, you are expected to know a lot about dealing with cases you are more familiar with. Also, you have acquired basic clinical skills such as professionalism, problem solving, and researching the literature, which you can apply to any case, regardless of the disorder.

4. **Inadequate supervision:** The American Speech-Language-Hearing Association requires that practicum experiences be supervised according to specific guidelines. For instance, assessments must be supervised in such a way that your supervisor watches 50% of your evaluation. In treatment, the requirement is 25% observation time. These, of course, are minimums, and many cases could easily benefit from 100% supervision if the case is complex and the student clinician is inexperienced. Some students report that they would like more supervision than they are receiving on a particular case and it frustrates them that their supervisor is not more involved. Certainly, most people would want the most supervision that they possibly could get, but you have to consider workload considerations and the ASHA guidelines. Adequate supervision may not be enough from your perspective, but if it meets ASHA guidelines and your supervisor is comfortable with it, that is the end of the story. Over years of working in university clinics we have seen many supervisors. Some supervise intensively and exceed ASHA guidelines. A *very few* are the subject of student complaints. For example, some students might say, "She's never around," or "I know she wasn't in the observation room at all this week," or "We only had 10 minutes for our supervisory conference and most of the time she talked about her dog." We are here to tell you that such instances are unacceptable for clinical supervisors and most do their job superbly. If, however, you are not satisfied with the amount or type of supervision you are given, the first step is to bring this up with the supervisor. Lay out your concerns in an organized and respectful fashion. For example, you might say, "I'm concerned that I have not gotten any written or verbal feedback on my performance for the past 3 weeks. We also have missed three supervisory conferences. I know you are busy, but I would appreciate your input so I can learn to be a better clinician." If no change occurs, it is important that you use whatever channels are available in your department to communicate this concern to the clinical director or department chairperson.

5. **Oppressive supervision:** In some cases, the supervisor is so involved in the treatment that the student has difficulty feeling "ownership" of the client. For example, a supervisor may frequently burst into the treatment room and "take over" the activity. Some of this behavior is beneficial under the goal of modeling good clinical skills, and you should be grateful for the

opportunity to observe. If, however, it happens too much and on activities that you already feel comfortable with, then you should voice this concern to your supervisor. Another example of a supervisor who is being too aggressive is when you are not able to participate in the goal setting for your client. When your supervisor tells you the goals, prescribes specific activities, outlines how you will keep track of treatment data, and does not allow an opportunity for student input, the learning experience is affected. Earlier, we stated that the student should have the opportunity to engage in problem solving, develop strategies for selecting goals, provide rationales, and have a role in planning. If the supervisor is telling you everything to do, it is essentially the supervisor doing therapy by proxy through the student. This is not an optimal learning experience. The student should be able to request a discussion of the treatment program and let the supervisor provide feedback about the student's ability to plan and execute the program.

6. **Personality conflicts with supervisor:** At its very base, the relationship between a supervisor and a practicum student is an interaction between two people. Although we stated earlier that it is the relationship between a teacher and a student, this does not exclude the fact that two individuals are interacting. Just as a student can have negative feelings toward a classroom teacher or a roommate, it is possible that in the more intensive relationship between the student and supervisor negative feelings can emerge as well. This is generally no one's fault, but just the inescapable reaction of two people who rub each other the wrong way. It can be very idiosyncratic and unfair. There is little to be done about this complaint because neither the student nor the supervisor is going to change his personality. So the most productive way to think about this is that you will have scores of supervisors, bosses, coordinators, teachers, and administrators who will be overseeing your work during your career. Although most of these people will be easy to get along with, there will always be a few who are not a perfect fit. Our best advice is to be philosophical about it and treat it as a learning experience. Getting along with difficult

people is a skill that will come in handy for your entire career, whether they are bosses, clients or coworkers. Try to minimize your contact time, avoid pushing any hot buttons, and be respectful of the person. As long as you perform your obligations as a student clinician in a professional and timely manner, you are doing what is required of a supervisee.

7. **Differing criteria for clinical writing among supervisors:** A major complaint of students is that various clinical supervisors have different criteria for writing reports. A student can write a report for one supervisor and receive compliments on report-writing ability. When those same phrases are used in a report for a different supervisor, they are deleted with a red pencil and the student is told the writing is unprofessional. It is true that supervisors have idiosyncratic views of how reports should be written. Although they agree on issues such as format and the use of professional terminology, there will always be unique aspects to what they prefer. The worst thing a student can do is to say, "I wrote it this way for Ms. Smith and she said it was correct." You have to decide, as the old country and western song says, "when to hold 'em and when to fold 'em." Arguing about inconsistencies among supervisors is almost always a losing strategy. The best thing to do is to find out from other students and the clinical records how a particular supervisor has approved writing in the past, and stick with that particular style. After you learn the idiosyncrasies of all your supervisors you can shift appropriately, and you have had the opportunity to learn many styles of writing. When you graduate, you can develop your own style, which will no doubt be an amalgamation of all your former clinical supervisors with your individual preferences.

8. **Differing criteria for grading among supervisors:** Just as classroom teachers differ in their grading methods, so do clinical supervisors. Students are aware that in some classes, most of the students earn As and Bs. On the other hand, there are classes where As and Bs are rare and there is a preponderance of average or lower grades. It is similar in the grading of clinical practicum, although we would suspect based

on our conversations with other university programs that grade inflation is especially prevalent in clinical practicum. Most students assume that they will earn an A or B in clinic, but a C is regarded almost as an F is viewed in classroom courses. We are not certain why this occurs in many programs, but it does. Nonetheless, even within the population of clinical supervisors, there are different grading styles; some are simply harder graders than others. In order to better understand the clinical grading system for an individual supervisor you can see that it is extremely important to discuss the variables you will be graded on at the outset of the semester. Do not be shy about asking what separates an A student in clinic from one who earns a B or a C. Focus on specific behaviors so that you can put your efforts into earning the grade that you desire. Also, do not underestimate the value of frequent conferences with the supervisor to ask for specific feedback on your performance in terms of a grade. Do not be afraid to ask, "If you had to give me a grade at this point, what would it be?" Also, query your supervisor about specific behaviors you need to change to attain a higher grade. Again, professional verbal communication is critical to resolving this issue.

9. **Supervisory conferences that run over time:** It is easy to lose track of time during supervisory conferences. Sometimes the student asks more questions than usual, or the supervisor needs extra time to explain a clinical technique that will be used in the next therapy session. Whatever the cause of running over the allocated time, this should be avoided if at all possible. Due to schedules, the supervisor has meetings, other cases to watch, or other students with whom to meet. Students have classes that abut with the supervisory conference and running over in the conference will make the student late for class. This is one reason why we recommended earlier that students become very organized about their questions and issues to raise in the conference setting. Supervisors, too, should be able to use the allocated time efficiently and not run over. If the problem becomes chronic, the supervisor will terminate the conference at the appropriate time and ask the student to become more organized. If the supervisor tends to keep the student late, the student needs to say, "I'm sorry, but I have a class this hour and I don't want to be late."

MISTAKES STUDENTS MAKE

1. **Complaining to other students:** One thing students have a tendency to do is voice their frustrations to other students in order to gain empathy and support. In most cases, this merely serves to escalate the frustration and spread it to other students. You can be certain that all you will get from your peers is support, sympathy, and validation of your complaint. The student says, "Ms. Paxton wants me to read *two articles* just to work with my client!" The other students say, "Wow, I can't believe she is doing that to you; we have so much to read for our classes. I'm glad I don't have her this semester." And so it escalates until the whole practicum student population is walking around with stifled outrage. Complaining just for the sake of complaining does not solve anything. Actually, when the supervisor assigned the readings, it should have been clear to the student why they were necessary. If it was not clear, then the student should ask the supervisor what points in particular should be attended to in the articles and how they will be integrated into the treatment. If you understand the purpose of the readings, and if the explanation makes sense, there is nothing to complain about, unless, of course, you just want to whine, which is not very productive.

2. **Not taking time to clarify how student and supervisor evaluations will be done:** As far back as Chapter 2 we mentioned the importance of discussing grading criteria at the outset of the clinical practicum experience with your supervisor. You should be aware of exactly which clinical behaviors are important, your responsibilities, and how you will be graded. If possible, you should obtain a sample copy of an evaluation/grading form that will actually be used in the grading process. There is no excuse for arriving at the end of the semester and saying,

"I didn't know that was important and I was being graded on it." Also, in almost every clinic, students are given the opportunity to evaluate the quality of clinical supervision that occurs during a semester. There is nothing wrong with discussing the behaviors that the supervisor will be "graded" on at the end of the term. If nothing else, it will bring to a conscious level in both the mind of the supervisor and the student what attributes are important in their practicum relationship.

3. **Failure to discuss the issue with the supervisor:** All the talking with students and other faculty members will not resolve a problem between your supervisor and you. It is always the best policy to go to your supervisor first to discuss any issue you are concerned about. This can be done in an organized and respectful manner, and in most cases the issue will be resolved in a positive way. Instead of wasting time talking to other people, go to your supervisor and say, "I was wondering if I might talk with you about a concern I have." We guarantee you that the supervisor will be "all ears" and engage you in a discussion to resolve your problem. Now, it may not always be resolved the way you would prefer, but at least you have aired the issue and will receive a more detailed explanation of the supervisor's point of view. In the case of reading articles mentioned above, the supervisor might say, "The articles will show you how to do three specific tasks with your client, how to gather treatment data, and provide a good rationale for organizing your treatment plan, which is due next week." You still may not like reading the articles, but you've got to admit, the supervisor has some pretty good reasons to ask you to read them.

4. **Copying written materials from prior reports without thinking:** While in clinical practicum in the university clinic, you will often be assigned to work with a client who received treatment for several previous semesters. This client might also have been supervised by the same clinical faculty member during that time. Some students think that an easy thing to do is to simply copy the recommendations from the last report and turn those into a treatment plan. Sometimes these are copied verbatim from the previous semester's treatment report. There are several problems with this approach. First of all, the client may have changed since the last semester, especially if there has been a long break between terms. A second problem might be that you have a new supervisor taking over the case who may not agree with the recommendations. A third difficulty is that the information in prior reports might be wrong. We have seen, for example, students copy the same case history information section on a client over and over for a string of semesters. In one particular case, three successive reports written by different students stated that the client had normal hearing, when in fact it had never been screened due to lack of child cooperation in the evaluation. The supervisor never caught the error and signed the reports with the students who perpetuated the mistake. It is difficult to keep up with every detail of a client when you are supervising 20 different people. Also, once something is written down in a report, it tends to be treated as fact. Finally, and most important, if you merely copy a series of recommendations or other report information, you have not really taken the opportunity to think about why goals were recommended or how assessment data were gathered. You have not gone through the process of problem solving but are just copying goals generated by someone else. Remember, part of the practicum experience is designed to help you learn to plan treatment in some principled way. Certainly, you should consider recommendations from the previous semester, but you should try to understand why they were made and come up with new considerations based on your knowledge from classroom work. In some cases, the supervisor may be ready to make some changes in the treatment program and your suggestions will be a breath of fresh air.

5. **Failure to take initiative:** Most students tend to do what they are told and not go "the extra mile." One way to really impress your supervisor is to come to a conference with some additional material that you have researched related to your client. This additional effort will be appreciated by most supervisors and show that you have a

commitment to the case. Even if the supervisor does not want to incorporate the new material, it is something you might use with other clients, and it has shown that you have initiative.

6. **Failure to progressively assume more clinical responsibility:** As illustrated in Figure 12–1, students should assume more clinical responsibility as they progress in practicum. Most supervisors will know where you are in terms of clinical development just by being aware of the cases you have worked with and the number of semesters of clinic you have completed. A major attribute the supervisor is looking for is your ability to apply your knowledge and previous experience to the current case. So if the student says, "I've worked with two other children at this level of language development. In those cases we developed a program like this (hands program to supervisor). I can modify this program with your input, or if you want to go a different direction, I would be happy to learn a new approach." Notice this shows that the student has ideas based on past experience and is willing to use them, modify them, or take a different direction. It shows confidence, a reasoned approach to the case, and assumption of responsibility.

7. **Not being punctual for meetings and assignment deadlines:** A critical aspect of running *any type of clinical program in any setting* is making sure clinical sessions are started and completed on time and that paperwork deadlines are met. One of the most certain paths to a lower grade is to ignore deadlines and clinic schedules. There is no excuse for this, and if it happens to you it is important to acknowledge your error and try to never let it reoccur.

8. **Saying you understand when you don't:** Occasionally in a conference you will be told by your supervisor to incorporate a new task into treatment, but you do not understand what it is, how to do it, or why it is important. Some students in this situation will just nod their head, scribble down some notes, and never ask for clarification. They hope that talking to other students will clarify the issue or looking through class notes will assist them in understanding. It is almost always a losing strategy to not admit when you

are clueless. It is completely appropriate to say, "I was with you until you mentioned incorporating distinctive features into the therapy. Can you explain that a bit more, or tell me exactly where I might read about it before next week?" At least in this case you will get a more detailed explanation or a reference that will help you to design your therapy.

9. **Becoming frustrated with lack of client progress:** Everyone knows when a client is not making progress: the client, the family, the clinician, and the supervisor. Sometimes, the lack of progress goes along with a very severe disorder. Other times, it is possible that the treatment approach must be adjusted to result in more progress. If you are seeing your client over and over again, and the treatment data are not showing any progress, then it is absolutely appropriate to ask your supervisor about this issue. You can say, "I've been working with John for 6 weeks now and he has not made any progress. Is this a typical pattern of response to therapy, or should we be thinking about changing our approach?" Chances are that the supervisor is just as frustrated as the student if the client is not making progress. If it is the case that this profile of client response is expected, the supervisor will tell you. If not, it is a good opportunity to rethink the approach and the supervisor will appreciate the chance to make adjustments. In this case, the student will be credited with being thoughtful and having initiative.

10. **Taking too much initiative when you are uncertain how to handle the situation:** Every student should be aware of his clinical limitations. If you have never done a procedure such as parent counseling, it would be inappropriate for you to engage in this without your supervisor's knowledge and consent. A good way to get into trouble is to come to a supervisory conference and say, "Oh, I counseled the parents on what to do at home for Charlie's stuttering." The supervisor might just indicate that such an occurrence is rather strange because the issue of a home program had never been discussed in conferences, and you have no experience with parent counseling. Always check with your supervisor before you engage in any procedure.

There no doubt are other communication issues and mistakes students can make with practicum supervisors. We have tried to give examples of common ones so the student can be proactive in interactions with clinical supervisors. As you can see, professional verbal communication is the medium by which problems with supervisors are confronted and solved. Keep those lines of communication open.

Appendices

Generator of Common Terms Used in Professional Communication*

The Person Receiving Services: client, patient, child, student, the child's first name, use of a pronoun (he, she) Mr., Ms., or Mrs. followed by surname, the family, caretaker, spouse (wife/husband).

The Person Providing Services: the (this) clinician, speech-language pathologist, examiner, interventionist, evaluator, assessor, therapist.

Clinical Activity Completed: Treatment, remediation, intervention, rehabilitation, assessment, examination, testing, appraisal, diagnostic evaluation, counseling, training, therapy.

Parameters of Communication Involved: Speech, communication, articulation, phonology, language, voice, fluency, hearing, swallowing.

Indicator of Disorder: Disorder, errors, abnormality, anomaly, deviation, difficulty, dysfunction, impairment, problem, disability, handicapping condition, deficit.

General "Professional Tone" Words:

Ability, abilities

Administer, administered

Appear, appears, appeared

Audiometric

Awareness

Adjustment

Affect (emotion)

Auditory acuity

Augmentative Communication

Baseline

Behavior

Caretaker

Causal

Clinical

Conduct, conducted

Consistent, consistency

Demonstrates, (ed)

Elderly

Environment

Evidence, evidences, evidenced

Exhibits

Feeding

Functional

Goal, goals

Hospitalization, hospitalized

Impression, impressions

Impact

Indicate, indicates, indicated

Intelligibility

Intonation

Judgment

Level of performance

Minimal

Neonatal

Bilingual

Case History

Characteristics, characterized

Competency

Congenital

Demonstrate

Effect

Eligibility, eligible

Etiology, etiological

Feedback

Exhibited

Follow-up

Generalize, generalizes generalized

Historically

Identify, identified, identification

Improve, improves, improved

Increase, increases, increased

Informant, informants

Interview

Inventory

Limited, limitations

Manifest, manifests, manifested

Multiple

Nature

*Adapted from Haynes, W. O., & Hartman, D. E. (1975). "The Agony of Report Writing: A New Look at an Old Problem." *Journal of the National Student Speech and Hearing Association, 3,* 7–15.

Nonstandardized

Objective, objectives
Occur, occurs, occurred
Oral
Outlook
Parent
Perform, performs, performed
Persistent
Prenatal
Predisposing factor

Production
Profound
Progressive
Project, projects, projected
Psychometric
Range
Refer, referral, referred

Reliable

Response
Sample, sampling, sampled
Significant
Skill, skills
State, states, stated
Symptom, symptoms
Target behavior, behaviors
Terminate, terminated
Unremarkable
Valid

Verbalize, verbalizes, verbalized
Vocalize, vocalizations, vocalized

Normative, norm-referenced
Observation
Onset
Organic
Parameter
Pediatric
Performance

Postoperative
Precipitating factor
Produce, produces, produced
Profile
Progress
Prognosis, prognostic
Prosody, prosodic

Rate
Reinforcement
Report, reports, reported
Respond, responds, responded
Reveal, reveals, revealed
Severity

Significantly
Standardized
Status
Symptomatology
Task, tasks

Toddler
Utterance, utterances
Variable, variability, varied
Verbalization, verbalizations

Selected General Terms in Child Language

Pragmatic
Topic manipulation
Morphology
Vocabulary

Repairs
Cohesion
Bound morphemes
Lexicon

Word retrieval
Syntactic
Gestural
Cognitive attainments
Communicative function
Comprehension

Caretaker

Literacy
Multiword
Reciprocity
Receptive

Semantic
Grammatical
Play
Communicative intent
Linguistic structures
Processing, processes, processed
Caretaker-child interaction
Figurative language
Narrative
Turn-taking
Expressive

Selected General Terms in Adult Language

Word retrieval
Executive function
Premorbid
Brain injury
Closed head trauma
CVA
Flaccid
Motor, motoric
Neurogenic
Activities of daily living
Status Post
Hemiparesis
Auditory Comprehension
Circumlocution

Word finding
Lesion
Bedside assessment
Head injury
Coma
Dementia
Paralysis
Paresis
Neuromuscular
TBI
Anomia
Neglect
Cognition

Selected General Terms in Voice Disorders

Resonance
Respiratory
Vocal
Voice
Phonatory
Vocal quality
Loudness
Acoustic
Breath, breathing
Glottal, glottal attack
Vocal hygiene
Optimal

Tracheoesophageal

Aerodynamic
Dysphonia
Aphonia
Phonation
Nasality
Pitch
Perceptual
Emission
Frequency
Abuse, misuse
Habitual
Velopharyngeal, velopharyngeal closure

Selected General Terms in Phonology

Phonological process
Production
Phoneme
Distinctive features
Phonetic context
Articulation
Omission
Disortion
Coarticulation,
    coarticulatory

Stimulability, stimulable
Phonetic placement
Phonemic
Phonological awareness
Misarticulation
Movement
Substitution
Syllable shape

Selected General Terms in Fluency

Disfluency, disfluencies,
    disfluent
Prolongation
Block
Overt
Interiorized
Filled pause
Rate
Timing device

Repetition

Hesitation
Covert
Exteriorized
Pause
Avoidance
Secondary behavior(s)
Adaptation

Consistency
Circumlocution

Struggle

Selected General Terms for Dysphagia

Consistency
Liquids
Chewing
Deglutition
Bolus
Transport
Regurgitation
Videofluroscopic
Cough
Thin
Ground
Solids
Thin/Thick
Oral transit
Nectar
Penetration
VSA
NPO

Aspiration
Saliva
Swallow
Airway
Duration
Feeding
Oral intake
Positioning
Gagging
Pureed
Chopped
Barium swallow
Pooling
Mechanical soft diet
Honey
Pudding
FEES
MBS

Sample of a University Clinic Diagnostic Report for Child Client Speech-Language Evaluation

Identifying Information:

Name: Mitchell Talon

D.O.B.: 4/6/98

Age: 13.1

Address: 12 Main Street
Auburn, AL 36830

D.O.E.: 05/27/2011

Telephone: (334) 345-6789

Parent: Vivian Talon

Clinicians: Jerome Hamilton

Summary

Mitchell is a 13-year-old male with an unremarkable medical history. He presents today with a mild language delay and moderate deficits in auditory processing, particularly in the area of memory and recall. He was compliant and interactive during the evaluation session. It is recommended that Mitchell attend therapy two times per week for a one-hour session to address the aforementioned deficits.

Case History/Background Information

Mitchell Talon is a 13-year-old male who was seen at the Auburn University Speech and Hearing Clinic (AUSHC) on May 27 for a formal speech and language comprehensive evaluation. He was accompanied to the evaluation by his mother, Vivian Talon, who served as the primary informant. He was referred for a language evaluation following a hearing evaluation and diagnosis of auditory processing disorder at AUSHC on April 25, 2011. It was specifically recommended to evaluate his auditory processing skills. Mitchell has a history of chronic ear infections. His mother reports concerns with processing directions from his teacher at school, which affects his grades. He also demonstrates difficulty with following multistep directions and memory tasks. His mother also noted that he often confuses words, such as "pacifically" for "specifically." In school and at home, he requires increased processing time and numerous repetitions in order to comprehend novel as well as familiar information. Mitchell's mother noted that she would like to start implementing written directions at school and at home. Academically, language arts are a weakness and math is a strength. Mitchell is very social and participates in various athletic activities. He is the middle child, with a younger brother and an older brother. He is not currently taking any medications. Mitchell has not received speech or language services in the past.

Voice/Fluency

Based on informal observation, Mitchell exhibits age and gender-appropriate pitch and voice quality. No episodes of stuttering were observed or reported.

Oral-Peripheral Exam

Based on a cursory examination, the structure and function of the oral mechanism are judged to be within functional limits.

Social/Pragmatics

Mitchell demonstrated typical interaction skills with the clinicians and exhibited appropriate eye contact. He was cooperative, attending well to activities and remaining engaged in tasks throughout the session. Mitchell exhibited proper topic maintenance skills and initiated and participated well in conversation.

Articulation

Based on informal assessment, Mitchell's articulation skills appear to be within normal limits; no sound errors were noted during the evaluation. He is judged to be 100% intelligible to familiar and unfamiliar listeners.

Language

Test of Auditory Processing Skill-3 (TAPS-3):

Due to reported concerns with auditory comprehension, the *Test of Auditory Processing Skill-3 (TAPS-3)* was administered. Areas assessed included number memory forward (the ability to retain simple sequences of auditory information), number memory reversed (the ability to retain and manipulate simple sequences of auditory information), word memory (the ability to retain and manipulate simple sequences of auditory information), sentence memory (the ability to retain details in sentences of increasing length and grammatical complexity), auditory comprehension (the ability to understand spoken information) and auditory reasoning (the ability to understand implied meanings, make inferences, or come to logical conclusions given the information in the sentence(s) presented).

Subtest	Raw Score	Scaled Score	Age Equivalent	Rating
Word Discrimination	30	9	7:6	Average
Phonological Segmentation	33	11	12:9	Average
Phonological Blending	9	3	5:6	Below Average
Number Memory Forward	15	7	7:3	Average
Number Memory Reversed	8	5	7:6	Below Average
Word Memory	13	5	5:7	Below Average
Sentence Memory	27	9	11:7	Average
Auditory Comprehension	26	10	12:7	Average
Auditory Reasoning	13	8	9:11	Average

	Sum of Scaled Scores	Index Standard Scores
Phonologic (word discrimination, phonological segmentation, phonological blending)	23	88
Memory (number memory forward, number memory reversed, word memory, sentence memory)	26	83
Cohesion (auditory comprehension, auditory reasoning)	18	95
Overall (all subtests)	67	88

The *TAPS-3* utilizes scaled scores that are based out of 20 with 10 being the mean and 7–13 indicating within normal limits. Any score below 7 indicates a deficit in the area tested when compared to age appropriate peers. Index Standard Scores are based out of 150 with a mean of 100 and a standard deviation of 15. This means that scores falling between 85–115 indicate abilities within normal limits. Any score below 85 is deemed below average when compared to same-age peers.

continues

Mitchell's performance indicates scores at or within normal limits on all subtests except phonological blending, number memory reversed, and word memory. He demonstrated the most difficulty with phonological blending and memory tasks. Mitchell's greatest strength is in phonological segmentation. He also demonstrated strengths in cohesion tasks, including auditory comprehension and reasoning. Mitchell's overall standard score for this test is 88, which falls within normal limits. However, his memory index score of 83 is outside the range of normality, and recall tasks are recommended in therapy to increase his processing skills.

The Token Test for Children-2

The Token Test for Children-2 (*TTFC-2*) primarily measures a child's comprehension of spoken language (also called Listening Comprehension) for children ages 3:0–12:11. There are 4 parts to the *TTFC-2*. Part 1 requires the child to follow one-step directions using all the tokens available (Large and small tokens of various colors; ("Touch the large blue circle"). Part 2 requires the child to follow 2 step directions using the Large Tokens ("Touch the white square and the yellow square"). Part 3 requires the child to follow 2-step directions using all the tokens ("Touch the large blue square and the small green circle"). Part 4 requires the child to follow complex directions using all the tokens ("Before touching the yellow circle, pick up the red square"). Mitchell's scores were as follows:

Subtest	Raw Score
Part 1	10
Part 2	10
Part 3	7
Part 4	11
Overall	38
Percentile Rank	39
Standard Score	96
Descriptive Rating	Average
Age Equivalent	9:6

The *TTFC-2* yields four types of scores: raw scores, standard scores, percentile ranks, and age equivalents. Raw scores refer to the actual number of correct responses in each subtest. The raw scores are combined to give an overall raw score. The overall raw score is then converted to a Standard Score to compare Mitchell's performance with other children of equal age. Standard scores indicate the distance of the raw score from the average of children of the same age. A standard score of 100 is considered the exact average for the person's age, with a standard deviation of 15 points.

Mitchell's standard score of 96 falls within the average range when compared to his same-age peers. He was quick to point to the tokens and showed little difficulty completing tasks. He did struggle more with the complex or multistep directions. The clinician also noticed that he consistently transposed the colors red and yellow throughout testing.

The Comprehensive Assessment of Spoken Language

The *Comprehensive Assessment of Spoken Language* (CASL) was administered to assess Mitchell's language abilities. The core subtests for ages 11–12 were administered, which include antonyms, grammatical morphemes, sentence comprehension, non-literal language, and pragmatic judgment. The CASL yields standard scores for each subtest, an overall standard score, percentile rank, normal curve equivalent, and stanine. A standard score of 100 is considered to be average, with a standard deviation of 15 points. This places the range of normality from 85 to 115.

Subtest	Raw Score	Standard Score
Antonyms	40	116
Grammatical Morphemes	20	83
Sentence Comprehension	15	97
Nonliteral Language	25	99
Pragmatic Judgment	53	92

Core Composite Scores	
Sum of Core Standard Scores	487
Standard Score	95
Percentile	37
Normal Curve Equivalent	43
Stanine	4

All of Mitchell's subtest standard scores fall within or above normal limits except for the grammatical morpheme score of 83. He demonstrated difficulty in this area, which was presented in the form of analogies. At times, he did not identify the correct word tense to appropriately fulfill the analogies. Mitchell's greatest strength was in antonyms, yielding a standard score of 116. His overall language standard score of 95 places him within normal limits.

Recommendations

It is recommended that Mitchell receive therapy at AUSHC at a frequency of one time a week for one hour. Therapy goals should focus on improving word recall, phonological blending, and following multistep directions. Prognosis is judged to be good based on high level of family support and Mitchell's compliance and willingness to work. It is also recommended that Mitchell receive a test of vision to assess for colorblindness.

Jerome Hamilton, B.A.
Graduate Clinician
cc: Vivian Talon

Laura Willis, MCD, CCC/SLP
Clinical Supervisor

Sample of a University Clinic Diagnostic Report for Adult Client

Identifying Information

Name: Michael Bradley

D.O.B.: 7/15/61

Spouse: Charlotte Bradley

Address: 580 Main Street
Notasulga, AL 36866

D.O.E.: 1/14/13

Age: 51

Telephone #: (334) 444-4444

Clinicians: Judy Jones
Ashley Adams

Summary

Michael Bradley is a 51-year-old male who attended Auburn University Speech and Hearing Clinic for a speech and language evaluation. His medical history is significant for a left hemisphere cerebrovascular accident (CVA). Results of the evaluation reveal that Mr. Bradley exhibits mild anomic aphasia, indicating that he has mild difficulties with naming and relatively preserved auditory comprehension. He also demonstrates a mild neurogenic stuttering disorder with blocks and part-word repetitions. Although Mr. Bradley exhibits a mild stuttering disorder and a mildly reduced rate, he is judged to be 100% intelligible to unfamiliar and familiar listeners. Mr. Bradley was observed to use mostly sentence fragments to communicate. There appeared to be no deficit with comprehension of concrete information during the evaluation. His vision was reported to be within functional limits, however, the audiological screening revealed a bilateral mild hearing loss. It should be noted that Mrs. Bradley reported that Mr. Bradley was having a "really good day," therefore, the results of this evaluation may not be typical of his every day function. It is recommended that Mr. Bradley enroll in therapy to address speech and language deficits resulting from his CVA.

Case History

Michael Bradley is a 51-year-old male who was referred by his neurologist, Dr. Frank Stanley, for a comprehensive speech and language evaluation. Mr. Bradley has received no prior speech therapy services. Mr. Bradley's wife, Charlotte Bradley, accompanied him to the evaluation and supplemented case history information. Mr. Bradley has a remarkable medical history, which includes high blood pressure, smoking, anxiety, alcohol abuse, and clinical depression. Mr. Bradley experienced a left hemisphere stroke on November 19, 2012. The most recent medical report from Mr. Bradley's doctor stated that while he is experiencing right hemiparesis, he is able to manage activities of daily living with supervision. Mrs. Bradley reported that since the strokes Mr. Bradley has had "a hard time remembering his words" and that "he talks slow." She also noted that he stutters, which was not present before the strokes. Mr. Bradley stated that he was most concerned with "getting his words out." Mrs. Bradley reported that when he experiences word-finding difficulty, he will typically abandon the attempt to communicate. Mr. Bradley denies any symptoms of oral or pharyngeal dysphagia. Mr. Bradley reported that his vision is within functional limits when he wears his glasses. Mr. Bradley is currently not working due to the residual effects of the stroke, but was previously employed by Steris as a machinist. At this time, Mr. Bradley is ambulatory and walks with a cane. They have three daughters that live at home, ranging from the ages of 13 years old to 18 years old.

Assessment Results

Language

The *Western Aphasia Battery-Revised (WAB-R)* was administered during the evaluation. It is designed to measure a patient's language function following a stroke. Linguistic skills assessed include speech content, fluency, auditory comprehension, repetition, naming, reading, and writing. Nonlinguistic skills (drawing, calculation, block design, and apraxia) were not measured due to client fatigue.

Results:

Spontaneous Speech Score: 19/20
During conversation, Mr. Bradley was observed to be able to answer questions accurately and appropriately. He responded in a timely manner to questions, however, mild anomia and blocks and sound prolongations were noted. During picture description, Mr. Bradley was able to state the main details of the picture but used primarily sentence fragments.

Auditory Verbal Comprehension Score: 9.05/10
Mr. Bradley was able to correctly answer all simple to complex yes/no questions with the exception of one complex question. No repetition was required.

Repetition Score: 8.4/10
Mr. Bradley was able to repeat words, phrases, and simple sentences, but did demonstrate difficulty when the sentence length was increased to 10 words due to anomia. No verbal apraxia was observed.

Naming and Word Finding Score: 8.2/10
Mr. Bradley was able to provide an appropriate response to complete a sentence for most trials. Errors noted were semantic paraphasias.

Aphasia Quotient: 89.3
Based on the above results of the WAB-R, Mr. Bradley exhibits Anomic Aphasia. The aphasia quotient is the summary value of the individual's aphasic deficit. Based on Mr. Bradley's aphasia quotient of 89.3, he has a mild aphasic deficit.

The supplemental test for the WAB-R, which assesses reading and writing, was attempted during the evaluation. The reading portion of the test was completed. The writing portion was attempted but unable to be completed due to client fatigue.

Results:

- Total Reading Score: 90/100
- Writing Upon Request: 6/6
- Writing Output: 7/34
- Writing to Dictation: 4.5/10
- Writing Dictated Words: 10/10
- Alphabet 12.5/12.5

Reading strengths observed include:

- Choosing the best word from a choice of four to complete a sentence
- Performing simple one-step commands

Reading weaknesses observed include:

- Performing multiple step commands

Writing strengths observed include:

- Writing name and address
- Writing dictated words
- Writing the entire alphabet

continues

Writing weaknesses observed include:

- Writing sentences about what is happening in a picture
- Writing a dictated sentence
- Prolonged and significantly increased response for all writing tasks

The results of the supplemental test indicate that Mr. Bradley has a mild reading impairment and a moderate writing impairment.

Articulation

No articulation errors, dysarthria, or verbal apraxia were noted during informal assessment throughout the evaluation. Mr. Bradley's intelligibility was judged to be 100% intelligible to an unfamiliar listener.

Voice/Fluency

Stuttering Severity Instrument-3 (SSI-3): The *SSI-3* assesses stuttering severity through evaluation of the frequency and duration of stuttering events as well as assessment of any physical concomitants that may accompany the stuttering event. For the assessment two speaking samples were obtained, one was obtained through informal conversation and the other was obtained by having Mr. Bradley read a passage aloud.

Results:

- Frequency: 14
- Duration: 8
- Physical Concomitants: 2
- Total Overall Score: 24

Frequency is measured using a reading task and a speaking task. The percentage of stuttered syllables is computed, and then converted into a task score. The task score for each speaking task is added together in order to determine the frequency score. The frequency score indicates the frequency of stuttering events in speech. The duration score is measured using the three longest stuttering events in seconds. The three durations are added and then divided by three to obtain an average duration. The average is then converted to a scale score. The physical concomitants score is based on observations of all of the speaking samples. The only observed physical concomitant demonstrated by Mr. Bradley was neck tension. The results of the scores in these three categories indicate that Mr. Bradley falls within the range of the 24–40-percentile rank for adults and demonstrate a mild stuttering severity. His rate was mildly decreased during volitional speech.

Hearing/Vision

Mr. Bradley's hearing was screened by the clinicians in the evaluation room using a portable audiometer. In his right ear, he was able to hear 1000 Hz at 35 dB, 2000 Hz at 30 dB, and 4000 Hz at 40 dB. In his right ear, he was able to hear 1000 Hz at 20 dB, 2000 Hz at 30 dB, and 4000 Hz at 40 dB. The results of the hearing screening indicate that Mr. Bradley has a mild hearing loss in both ears. Mr. Bradley responded to speech at normal levels during the evaluation.

Mr. Bradley's vision was reported to be within functional limits and no visual acuity abnormalities were noted during the evaluation.

Oral Motor Exam

The Oral-Facial Examination Form was used to examine Mr. Bradley's oral motor functions including range of motion, strength, and coordination. Mr. Bradley's facial, lingual, labial, dental, and palatal movements, symmetry, and strength were judged to be within normal limits.

Recommendations/Prognoses

It is recommended that Mr. Bradley enroll in therapy to address speech and language deficits resulting from a left hemisphere CVA. It is also recommended that a comprehensive audiological evaluation be scheduled to assess Mr. Bradley's hearing abilities.

Therapy should focus on the following areas:

1. Establishing use of strategies to decrease disfluencies at the phrase and simple sentence level
2. Written language at the sentence level
3. Reading comprehension at a moderate level of difficulty
4. Complex level expressive tasks to decrease anomia
5. Establishing use of circumlocution when necessary
6. Other goals as appropriate per ongoing assessment

Prognosis for decreasing disfluencies at the phrase/simple sentence level is good due to motivation, self-awareness, and length of time post-onset. Mr. Bradley's prognosis for learning compensatory strategies for anomia, prognosis for comprehending moderate level written sentences and writing at the simple sentence level is fair to good. Positive prognostic indicators include intact cognition, self-awareness for errors, motivation, attention, and preserved auditory comprehension.

Madeline Moates, M.C.D, CCC-SLP
Speech-Language Pathologist

Judy Jones B.S.
Graduate Clinician

Ashley Adams B.S.
Graduate Clinician

APPENDIX D

Example of a Communication Addendum from a Medical Facility

COMMUNICATION ASSESSMENT
ADDENDUM

☐ Initial   ☐ Re-eval   ☐ D/C _____

ADDRESSOGRAPH

SEVERITY RATING/FIM SCORE	*Use these ratings on lines below.*
7 = *WFL*	*100%*
6 = *WFL/Assistive Device or Extra Time*	*Minimal Extra Time*
5 = *Occasional Difficulty*	*90% Requires Assistance <10% of time*
4 = *Minimally Impaired*	*75-90%*
3 = *Moderately Impaired*	*50-74%*
2 = *Maximally Impaired*	*25-45%*
1 = *Profoundly Impaired*	*0-24%*

NT = Not Tested
N/A = Not Assessable

AUDITORY COMPREHENSION: ___ Overall Severity Rating
____ Body Part Identification
____ Familiar Object I.D.
____ Yes / No Question:
　　____ Simple (basic needs/biographical info)
　　____ Complex
Directions:
　　____ 1 Step
　　____ 2 Step
　　____ 3 Step
____ Comprehends Simple Conversational Discourse
____ Comprehends Brief Narrative Discourse
　　(familiar content)
____ Right / Left Directions

READING COMPREHENSION: ___ Overall Severity Rating
Rate Each Area.
____ Word
____ Phrase
____ Sentence
____ Paragraph
____ Functional Reading Tasks
____ Other _____
_____
_____
_____

PRAGMATICS: ___ Overall Severity Rating
Rate Each Area.
____ Eye Contact
____ Initiation of Topic
____ Turn Taking
____ Topic Maintenance

HEARING SKILLS: ☐ Impaired ____ ☐ Aided ____ ☐ WFL
Comments:

VISUAL SKILLS: ☐ Impaired ____ ☐ Aided ____ ☐ WFL
Comments:

VOICE (check) ☐ Trach ___ Overall Severity Rating
Vocal Quality: ☐ WFL ☐ Strained/Harsh ☐ Breathy
　　　　　　 ☐ Wet ☐ Other _____
Breath Support: ☐ WFL ☐ Shallow ☐ Other _____
Volume: ☐ WFL ☐ Too Soft ☐ Too Loud
Pitch: ☐ WFL ☐ Monotone ☐ Sing Song

INTELLIGIBILITY: ___ Overall Severity Rating
Word _____ Phrase/sentence _____ Conversation _____

EXPRESSION: ___ Overall Severity Rating
____ Yes / No Response (verbal/gestural)
____ Gestural Communication
____ Automatic/Recitation Speech
____ Responsive Naming
____ Spontaneous/Functional Word Production
____ Sentence Formulation
____ Conversation _____
_____

WRITTEN EXPRESSION: ___ Overall Severity Rating
Hand Dominance ☐ R ☐ L　　Hand Utilized ☐ R ☐ L
Content:
Name _____ Word _____ Sentence _____ Functional Tasks _____
Legibility:
Name _____ Word _____ Sentence _____ Functional Tasks _____

BEHAVIORAL OBSERVATION: *(Check if apply)*
____ Perseveration
____ Sound/Word Substitutions
____ Circumlocutions
____ Confused/confabulatory Language/Jargon
____ Neglect L / R
____ Delayed Response Formulation
____ Verbosity/tangential
____ Delayed Auditory Processing Time
____ Limb Apraxia
____ Other _____

MOTOR SPEECH:
Rate Each Area.
Fluency/Disorder ☐ WFL ☐ Min. ☐ Mod. ☐ Severe ☐ Profound
Dysarthria ☐ WFL ☐ Min. ☐ Mod. ☐ Severe ☐ Profound
Apraxia (oral/verbal) ☐ WFL ☐ Min. ☐ Mod. ☐ Severe ☐ Profound

Comments: _____
_____
_____
_____
_____
_____
_____
_____
_____
_____
_____
_____
_____
_____
_____
_____

Signature/Title/Date/Time	**Signature/Title/Date/Time**

Appendix D. Example of a Communication Addendum from a Medical Facility

Example of a Cognitive Addendum from a Medical Facility

COGNITIVE ASSESSMENT ADDENDUM

☐ Initial   ☐ Re-eval   ☐ D/C _____

ADDRESSOGRAPH

SEVERITY RATING/FIM SCORE   *Use these ratings on lines below.*

7 = *WFL*	*100%*	NT = Not Tested
6 = *WFL/Assistive Device or Extra Time*	*Minimal Extra Time*	N/A = Not Assessable
5 = *Occasional Difficulty*	*90% Requires Assistance <10% of time*	
4 = *Minimally Impaired*	*75-90%*	
3 = *Moderately Impaired*	*50-74%*	
2 = *Maximally Impaired*	*25-45%*	
1 = *Profoundly Impaired*	*0-24%*	

LEVEL OF ALERTNESS: (Check One)
____ Alert/focused
____ Alert/unfocused/inattentive
____ Lethargic/somnolent
____ Unresponsive

PROBLEM SOLVING/REASONING: ___ Overall Severity Rating
____ Simple, non-verbal reasoning
____ Complex, non-verbal reasoning
____ Simple verbal reasoning
____ Abstract/complex verbal reasoning
____ Calculation

ATTENTION: ____ Overall Severity Rating
____ Sustained attention to task in 1:1 environment (greater than 3 minutes)
____ Selective attention in distracting environment
____ Divided attention in distracting environment
____ Sustained Level II (mental control)
____ Alternating

ORIENTATION: ____ Overall Severity Rating
____ Person
____ Place (building, city, state)
____ Time (year, month, day, date)
____ Situation

MEMORY: ____ Overall Severity Rating
____ Recalls biographical information

	Verbal	Visual
Immediate Memory	_____	_____
Short Term Memory	_____	_____
Long Term Memory	_____	_____
Procedural Memory	_____	_____

EXECUTIVE FUNCTION: _____ Overall Severity Rating
____ Initiation
____ Goal Setting
____ Organization
____ Planning/Decision Making
____ Self Monitoring
____ Time Management

INSIGHT: ____ Overall Severity Rating
____ Demonstrates awareness of current limitations/deficits
____ Expresses need for assistance
____ Demonstrates ability to compensate for deficits

SAFETY AWARENESS: ____ Overall Severity Rating
____ Demonstrates awareness of need for safety precautions during functional situation
____ Demonstrates use of safety precautions during functional situation

REFERRAL/TX SECTION: (Check all that apply)
____ Behavioral Program
____ Formal Neuropsych Evaluation
____ Referral for Treatment of Above Deficits
____ Other

BEHAVIORAL/MOTIVATION: (Check all that apply)
____ Impulsive   ____ Disinhibited
____ Agitated/Aggressive   ____ Flat Affect
____ Perseveration   ____ Poor Initiation
____ Other

COMMENTS/OTHER: _____
_____
_____
_____
_____
_____
_____
_____
_____
_____
_____

Signature/Title/Date/Time	**Signature/Title/Date/Time**

Revised 4/08   Page 1 of 1   ©2010 HealthSouth Corporation   326 Cognitive Addendum
                                                              REORDER # HLS-FM-384033-01

Appendix E. Example of a Cognitive Addendum from a Medical Facility

Example of a Dysphagia Addendum from a Medical Facility

REGIONAL
REHABILITATION HOSPITAL

DYSPHAGIA ASSESSMENT ADDENDUM

☐ Initial ☐ Re-eval ☐ D/C _____ ADDRESSOGRAPH

CURRENT DIET: _____
SWALLOWING HISTORY: _____
_____

PREVIOUS MBS: ☐ YES ☐ NO DATE/RESULTS: _____
_____

GENERAL OBSERVATIONS:

Patient Positioning:	☐ Upright In Chair/Bed	☐ Other _____	
Alertness:	☐ Alert	☐ Lethargic	☐ Inconsistent
Behavior:	☐ Distractible	☐ Noncompliant	☐ Impulsive
Commun./Cognitive Status:	☐ Memory WFL	☐ Follows Simple Commands	
	☐ Verbalizes Needs	☐ Receptive Language Deficits	
	☐ Expressive Aphasia	☐ Apraxia	

Oral Motor
Labial	☐ Adequate	☐ Inadequate _____
Lingual	☐ Adequate	☐ Inadequate _____
Dry Swallow	☐ Adequate	☐ Inadequate _____
Cough/Throat Clear	☐ Adequate	☐ Inadequate _____
Facial Symmetry	☐ L / R Facial Droop	☐ Hypertonicity/Hypotonicity
Dentition	☐ Full Dentures	☐ Partial Dentures ☐ Missing Teeth ☐ Malocclusion
Trach:	☐ No ☐ Yes	Type/Size _____
(During Exam)	☐ Inflated ☐ Deflated ☐ Capped ☐ Uncapped	
Vocal Quality:	☐ Wet ☐ Hoarse ☐ Breathy	☐ Other

Check, if apply:	W F L	Difficulty Chewing L / R / B	Pocketing L / R / B	Increased Oral Transit Time	Bolus Formation Difficulty	Coughing	Change In Vocal Quality	Delayed Swallowing	Decreased Laryngeal Evaluation	Other
Puree										
Ground										
Mechanical Soft										
Chopped										
Regular										
Thin Liquid										
Nectar Thick										
Honey Thick										

STRATEGIES - FOODS:
☐ Place Food in R / L Side	☐ Discourage Talking While Eating	☐ Slow Rate
☐ Chin Down	☐ Lingual Sweep	☐ Tilt Head Back
☐ Encourage Chewing	☐ Multiple Swallow	☐ Alternate Food/Liquid
☐ Small Bites	☐ Quiet Environment	☐ N/A
☐ Check For Pocketing	☐ Turn/Tilt Head L /R	
☐ Other:_____		

STRATEGIES - LIQUID:
☐ Spoon Only	☐ No Straw
☐ From Cup	☐ Use Straw
☐ Small Sips	☐ Turn / Tilt Head L /R
☐ Chin Down	☐ N/A
☐ Multiple Swallow	
☐ Other:_____	

ADDITIONAL ASSESSMENT/CONSULTATIONS:
☐ Instrumental Assessment _____	☐ Dietician Consultation	☐ Oral Motor Regime
☐ Follow-up Clinical Assessment on _____	☐ Self Feeding Referral	☐ Speech / Language
☐ Dysphagia Therapy	☐ Other _____	Evaluation & Treat

SUMMARY: _____
_____
_____

Dysphagia: ☐ Oral ☐ Oropharyngeal ☐ Pharyngeal ☐ Pharyngoesophageal ☐ No Therapy Indicated

RECOMMENDATIONS:
Diet Consistency: Solids: _____ Liquids: _____ NPO: _____
Medications: ☐ Non Oral ☐ Crushed ☐ Liquid ☐ Whole ☐ Other _____
Level of Supervision: ☐ 1 - 1 by _____ ☐ Feeding Group ☐ Tray Setup ☐ Intermittent ☐ None

Signature/Title/Date/Time	Signature/Title/Date/Time

Appendix F. Example of a Dysphagia Addendum from a Medical Facility

Example of an Eligibility Form Used in Public Schools

NOTICE AND ELIGIBILITY DECISION REGARDING
SPECIAL EDUCATION SERVICES

Student's Name:				Page		of	
Date this report was given or sent to parent (student at age 19)							

Check One:	[ ]	Initial Eligibility		[ ]	Reevaluation

Vision Screening			Hearing Screening		
Date		Result	Date		Result

Area of Assessment:	
Date:	
Assessment:	
Standard Scores (Total):	
Other Scores:	

Date:	
Assessment:	
Standard Scores (Total):	
Other Scores:	

Date:	
Assessment:	
Standard Scores (Total):	
Other Scores:	

Area of Assessment:	
Date:	
Assessment:	
Standard Scores (Total):	
Other Scores:	

Date:	
Assessment:	

Appendix G. Example of an Eligibility Form Used in Public Schools *continues*

Standard Scores (Total):	
Other Scores:	

Date:	
Assessment:	
Standard Scores (Total):	
Other Scores:	

Student's Name:		Page		of	

Area of Assessment:	

Date:	
Assessment:	
Standard Scores (Total):	
Other Scores:	

Date:	
Assessment:	
Standard Scores (Total):	
Other Scores:	

Date:	
Assessment:	
Standard Scores (Total):	
Other Scores:	

Area of Assessment:	

Date:	
Assessment:	
Standard Scores (Total):	
Other Scores:	

Appendix G. *continues*

Date:	
Assessment:	
Standard Scores (Total):	
Other Scores:	

Date:	
Assessment:	
Standard Scores (Total):	
Other Scores:	

Final Completion Date of <u>ALL</u> Evaluations: _____

Student's Name:		Page		of	

SLD ONLY SECTION – For each option checked below, include documentation of a specific learning disability in the assessment section of this report.

[ ] Option 1: Response(s) to Intervention.

[ ] Option 2: Pattern of strengths and weaknesses.

[ ] Option 3: Severe Discrepancy (SD) documentation.

A. If using the predicted achievement model (regression to the mean effective 7/1/98):					
IQ score:					
			PA	- OA	= SD
Predicted Achievement (PA) score:					
Obtained Achievement (OA) score(s)			PA	- OA	= SD
determined one of two ways:					
One Achievement Test			(SD must be 16 points or greater for all ages)		
Total test score					
OR					
Two Composites OR Two Subtests					
Scores from two different achievement tests that measure the same deficit skill area (i.e., Composite Reading scores from two different tests; Subtest Calculation scores from two different tests)					
Severe discrepancy (SD) between ability and achievement: [ ] YES [ ] NO					

Appendix G. *continues*

B. If using the simple standard score method (only for students identified before July 1, 1998):

Complete for all students suspected of SLD, regardless of option(s) chosen above.

1. For educationally relevant <u>behaviors noted during the classroom observation(s)</u> and educationally relevant medical findings (if any), please refer to page(s) ____ of this report.

2. Student behavior or difficulty that affects his/her academic functioning:

3. The following factors have been ruled out as the <u>primary cause</u> of the impairment (all must be considered and checked to qualify for SLD):

   [ ] Environmental/Cultural/Economic Concerns   [ ] Visual/Hearing
   Disabilities   Disabilities

   [ ] Intellectual Disability   [ ] Emotional Disability   [ ] Motor Disabilities

Student's Name:		Page	of

ELIGIBILITY DECISION

ELIGIBLE: [ ] YES   [ ] NO
AREA OF DISABILITY: _____ ____

___

If the selected area of disability is Multiple Disabilities, list at least two disability areas for which the student is eligible.

_____

Explanation (if needed):

Complete for all students:

Was lack of appropriate instruction in math and/or reading, including the essential components of reading instruction **(as defined in section 1208(3) of the Elementary and Secondary Education Act of 1965)** or limited English proficiency <u>the</u> determining factor in the decision?   [ ] YES [ ]
NO
(See documentation included in this report.)

Description of other options considered And why they were rejected

---

Check One: Eligibility Committee [ ]   **IEP Team** [ ]

I **AGREE** with the conclusions written in this report.		
Position	**Signature**	**Date**
Parent		
Parent		
General Education Teacher		
Special Education Teacher		
LEA Representative		
Someone Who Can Interpret The Instructional Implications Of The Evaluation Results		

Appendix G. *continues*

Student		
Other		

I **DO NOT AGREE** with the conclusions written in this report. The attached statement represents my conclusions in this area.

Position	Signature	Date

My signature below verifies that if you require notice and an explanation of your rights in your native language, the LEA/agency has accommodated you to ensure your understanding. You are fully protected under the rights addressed in your copy of the *Special Education Rights* document. You may access another copy of your rights at www.alsde.edu. Once in the Web site, select Sections/Special Education/Forms. If you cannot access the Web site and want another copy of your rights, have any questions, or wish to arrange a conference, please contact:

Name:		Telephone:	

Signature of Education Agency Official

Appendix G. *continued*

Example of a University Clinic Daily Treatment Plan

Daily Treatment Plan

Client: Kevin White
Clinician: R. Smith
Disorder: Language

File Number: 00-123-98
Supervisor: Haynes
Date: 1-13-13

Objectives and Procedures

Short-term Objective 1: The client will spontaneously produce 30 single words or word approximations in order to request, label or comment during a thirty-minute session.

> **Procedure**: The clinician and client will engage in a variety of structured play activities using high interest toys such as farm animals, Mr. Potato Head and bubbles. The clinician will structure the session to facilitate the client's need to request items or activities of interest. A choice may be provided as a cue if necessary. The client will be reinforced by receiving the item or activity he requested.

Short-term Objective 2: The client will follow one-step commands during structured play activities in 75% of opportunities during a thirty-minute session.

> **Procedure**: During structured play, the clinician will prompt the client with questions such as "Put the cow in the barn," "Put the top on the play-doh," and "Give me the ball." If cues are required, the stimulus will be repeated and then the clinician will model the desired action.

Example of a Speech Daily Treatment Form from an Acute Care Hospital

EAMC(Location: REN ; 4122 ; A)

DOB / AGE / SEX: 04/20/57 55 Years Female

Admitting Physician: ███████████

Admission Date / MRN / Financial Num: 09/21/12 590370 1226500028

Speech Treatment Daily Form

09/26/12 12:50 pm Performed by ███████████

Entered on 09/26/12 01:00 pm

General Info

Affect/Behavior: Calm, Cooperative

Goals

Speech Treatment Goals Grid

	ST Goal 1	ST Goal 2	ST Goal 3
Speech/Language Goal	Pt will answer yes/no questions with 80% accuracy.	Pt will follow commands with 80% accuracy.	Pt will imitate phonemes and simple words with 70% accuracy.
Speech Goal Set	09/25/12	09/25/12	09/25/12

	ST Goal 4
Speech/Language Goal	Pt will perform identification tasks with 80% accuracy.
Speech Goal Set	09/25/12

Todays Progress Toward Goals Grid

	ST Goal 1	ST Goal 2	ST Goal 3
Todays Progress Toward Goal ST	Pt answered 4/7 yes no questions with moderate to heavy cueing.	Pt followed commands with 65% accuracy independently, increasing to 100% accuracy with heavy cueing.	Pt imitated /pa/ in 1/4 trials with heavy cueing.

	ST Goal 4
Todays Progress Toward Goal ST	Pt identified 4/7 body parts independently, increasing to 100% with moderate cueing.

Justification for Skilled Speech Service: S/p CVA

Plan

Speech Current Plan: Continue current POC

Speech/Language Treatment Frequency: Six times a week

Speech/Language Treatment Planned Dur: Three weeks

Planned Speech/Language Treatment Tech: Speech/Language/Communication Treatment

Treatment

Speech Treatment Provided this Date: Pt was awake and alert when S. Th. arrived. Pt identified several body parts independently and identified others when given a model. Pt followed most commands independently but when asked to point to something the pt required heavy cueing to complete the task. This was done by having the pt follow the therapist's finger through the air to point to the items. Yes/no questions required imitation and a physical cue to accomplish head nodding for yes for 4/7 trials. Continue to work on establishing a reliable nod for yes and then move to establish side to side head movement for no. The pt was able to imitate the syllable /pa/ one time with heavy verbal cueing and multiple models. In other trials the pt was unsuccessful but made attempts at moving her lips into position to produce the /p/. S. Th. will continue to follow.

Charges

Cognitive Skills Development Minutes ST: 0 minute(s)

Speech/Language/Voice/Auditory Trea Min: 25 minute(s)

Speech/Language/Voice/Auditory Trea Char: Yes

Appendix I. Example of Speech Daily Treatment Form from an Acute Care Hospital

Selected Acronyms Used in School Settings

ADA — *Americans with Disabilities Act*

ADD — Attention Deficit Disorder

ADHD — Attention Deficit Hyperactivity Disorder

APR — Annual Performance Report

AT — Assistive Technology

AUT — Autism

AYP — Adequate Yearly Progress

BIP — Behavioral Intervention Plan

CRS — Children's Rehabilitation Services

CEIS — Coordinated Early Intervening Services

DB — Deaf-Blindness

DIBELS — Dynamic Indicators of Basic Early Literacy Skills

DPH — Due Process Hearing

ED — Emotional Disability

eGAP — Electronic Grant Application Process

EI — Early Intervention

ELL — English Language Learners

ELPP — Early Learning Progress Profile

ESA — Educational Service Agency

ESY — Extended School Year

FAPE — Free Appropriate Public Education

FBA — Functional Behavioral Assessment

GEP — Gifted Education Plan

GT — Gifted

HI — Hearing Impairment

IAES — Interim Alternative Educational Setting

ID — Intellectual Disability

IEP — Individualized Education Program

IFSP — Individualized Family Service Plan

LEA — Local Education Agency

LEP — Limited English Proficiency

LRE — Least Restrictive Environment

MD — Multiple Disabilities

NCLB — *No Child Left Behind Act of 2001*

OHI — Other Health Impairment

OI — Orthopedic Impairment

O&M — Orientation and Mobility

OSEP — Office of Special Education Programs

OT — Occupational Therapy/ Therapist

PBS — Positive Behavioral Supports

PST — Problem Solving Team

PT — Physical Therapy/ Therapist

Selected Medical Abbreviations Used in Documentation

A—assistance

ADL—activities of daily living

ARDS—adult respiratory distress

AX—assessment

△—change

b.i.d.—two times a day

BP—blood pressure

c̄—with

CAD—coronary artery disease

c/o—complains of

COPD—chronic obstructive pulmonary disease

CVA—cerebrovascular accident

↓—decreased

d/c—discharge

DM—diabetes mellitus

DNR—do not resuscitate

DVT—deep vein thrombosis

Dx—diagnosis

GERD—gastroesophageal reflux disease

h/o—history of

H&P—history and physical examination

HTN—hypertension

Hx—history

ICH—intercranial hemorrhage

↑—increased

L, lt—left

Max—maximum

MBS—modified barium swallow

MCA—middle cerebral artery

Min—minimum

Mod—moderate

MRI—magnetic resonance imaging

NG—nasogastric

NPO—nothing per oral

O—oriented (Ox3)

OMEs—oral motor exercises

PE—pulmonary embolism

PEG—percutaneous endoscopic gastrostomy

p.o.—by mouth

POC—plan of care

PRN—per necessary, or when needed

Pt—patient

R, rt—right

R/O—rule out

ROM—range of motion

q.d.—each day

SOB—shortness of breath

s/p—status post

s/s—signs/symptoms

t.i.d.—three times daily

Tx—thearpy

s̄—without

WNL—within normal limits

y/o—year old

VSA/VFSS—videofluoroscopic swallowing assessment

Example of an Individualized Family Service Plan (IFSP)

INDIVIDUALIZED FAMILY SERVICE PLAN

*Date: _____

*Type of meeting: ☐ Interim IFSP ☐ Initial IFSP ☐ Annual ☐ Review

| *Child's Name: | *Date of Birth: | ☐ *Male ☐ *Female |

Parent/Foster Parent/Guardian/Family Member (circle one)

*Name	
*Address	
*City	*State	*Zip
*Phone (day)	(Evening)
*Primary Language	

Parent/Guardian/Family Member (circle one)

*Name	
*Address	
*City	*State	*Zip
*Phone (day)	(Evening)
*Primary Language	

*Surrogate Parent: _____ *Phone: _____

*Address: _____

*Service Coordinator/Program: _____ *Phone: _____

*Address: _____

*Physician/Health Care Provider: _____ *Phone: _____

*Address: _____

*School District: _____ Contact Person/Phone: _____

*Recommended school district referral date, no later than: _____
(Refer the child any time after the 2nd birthday. The decision to refer must be made no later than age 2 1/2)   _____ date
☐ *Check if release to LEA (form 3-3) is on file

*Denotes part of the electronic record   _____ date
☐ *Check if referral to LEA (form 3-8) is on file

Connecticut Birth to Three Form 3-1 (Revised 7/1/06)

Appendix L. Example of an Individualized Family Service Plan (IFSP). (Used with Permission from Connecticut Birth to Three System.) *continues*

Child's Name: _____ DOB: _____ Date: _____

SECTION I. SUMMARY OF CHILD'S PRESENT ABILITIES, STRENGTHS, AND NEEDS

1. Indicate the dates and types of evaluation or assessment report, which were used to develop this plan:

_____

2. Summarize below additional observations by family and other team members of the child's abilities, strengths, and needs in daily routines. Areas to include:

● What are your child's likes and dislikes?   ● Bathing, feeding, dressing, toileting – Adaptive/Self help skills
● What are your child's frustrations?   ● Thinking, reasoning and learning – Cognitive skills
● How does your child spend his/her day?   ● Moving, hearing, vision, health – Physical development
                                              ● Feelings, coping, getting along with others – Social/Emotional development
                                              ● Understanding, communicating with others and expressing self with others – Communication skills

_____

_____

_____

_____

_____

_____

_____

_____

_____

_____

_____

(Attach additional pages as needed)

Connecticut Birth to Three Form 3-1 (Revised 7/1/06)

Appendix L. *continues*

Child's Name: _____ DOB: _____ Date: _____

SECTION II. SUMMARY OF FAMILY'S CONCERNS, PRIORITIES, AND RESOURCES AS THEY RELATE TO ENHANCING THEIR CHILD'S DEVELOPMENT - Family Outcome

1. Information about our family for the IFSP: (Suggestions)

- Things we like to do as a family
- Who is part of our family?
- Important events that have occurred

- People and agencies we find helpful.
- Our family's strengths in meeting our child's needs.
- How our child's special needs affect our family

2. What would be helpful for our family in the months and year ahead? (Family Outcome)

3. What assistance or information will we need to achieve this outcome? (Strategies)

SECTION III. OTHER SERVICES THAT ARE IN PLACE OR ARE NEEDED

Services such as medical, recreational, religious, social and other child related services, not covered by the CT Birth to Three System, that contribute to this plan.

Resource/Program/Support Service	✓ If Needed	Payment Source

Connecticut Birth to Three Form 3-1 (Revised 7/1/06)

Confidential Document

Appendix L. *continues*

190

Child's Name: _____ DOB: _____ Date: _____

SECTION IV. PLAN FOR TRANSITION FROM THE BIRTH TO THREE SYSTEM TO PRESCHOOL SPECIAL EDUCATION OR OTHER APPROPRIATE SERVICES

1. Information that would be helpful for our child and family to plan for the future. •Community program options •LEA information •Referral process • Rights and responsibilities •Parent training •Visiting community programs •Adaptive equipment •Transportation •Time with other children • Information sharing.

2. What are the next steps?	Who will be involved:	Date to be completed:

After the initial IFSP meeting, this plan may only be modified at an IFSP periodic review meeting or annual IFSP meeting

Connecticut Birth to Three Form 3-1 (Revised 7/1/06)

Appendix L. continues

Child's Name: _____ DOB: _____ Date: _____

SECTION V. OUTCOME #____

What we want is: _____

What is happening now: _____

What are the next steps (objectives) to reach this outcome?

	Expected timeframe for reaching objective

Strategies: methods for working on this outcome during your child and family's daily activities and routines

	People who will be involved

(Attach additional pages as needed)

Appendix L. *continues*

SECTION VI. EARLY INTERVENTION SERVICES AND SUPPORTS

*What is going to happen (including assistive technology)	*Delivered by: (Discipline responsible)	*Location Code	*How Often	*How Long	*Start Date	*End Date

☐ Check here if additional pages are attached to list or clarify the services being provided or the schedule of services.

Primary service location codes: 1=home 2=setting designed for typical children 3=hospital (inpatient) 4=residential facility 5=service provider office 6=setting designed for children with delays 7=other

☐ *Check if any early intervention service cannot be achieved satisfactorily in a natural environment and attach a justification for each service.

Informed Consent by Parents. Check and sign below:

1. _____ I understand my rights under this program and received a written copy of *Parent Rights Under IDEA Part C* **and**

2a. _____ I give permission to carry out this Individualized Family Service Plan as written.

or

2b. _____ I do not accept this Individualized Family Service Plan as written, however I do give permission for the following services to begin:

Services are paid for by the Birth to Three System unless otherwise indicated:
Service Coordinator/ Discipline/ Program Name/phone #:
Service Coordination is provided to all families at least monthly and is most often part of the early intervention visit

Parent Signature _____ Date _____

Parent Signature _____ Date _____

I have reviewed this Individualized Family Service Plan, which is based in part on an evaluation in all areas of development. I confirm the appropriateness of the diagnosis(es) as stated by the diagnostic (ICD-9) code and the recommendations for the treatment services as they are written.

Physician Signature: _____ LIC#: _____ *Date: _____

*Print Name: _____ *ICD-9 Code(s) _____

*Denotes part of the electronic record

Connecticut Birth to Three Form 3-1 (Revised 7/1/06)

Appendix L. *continues*

Child's Name: _____ DOB: _____ Date: _____

SECTION VII. IFSP TEAM MEMBERS

The following individuals have participated in the development of the IFSP and/or will assist in its implementation. There will be ongoing verbal communication between the IFSP team members listed below to assist in the implementation of the IFSP.

Name	Relationship	Phone	Method of participation

Meeting Notes: (discussion, specific scheduling issues, and any other issues)

Connecticut Birth to Three Form 3-1 (Revised 7/1/06)

Appendix L. *continues*

Section R-1: Individualized Family Service Plan (IFSP) Review: Outcomes

☐ Periodic review
☐ Annual review

Child's Name: _____ DOB: _____ Review Date: _____

Date of IFSP being reviewed: _____ Reason for review: _____

Outcome #	Outcome(s)	Progress towards reaching *family* outcomes	Status

Outcome #	Outcome(s)	Progress towards reaching *child* outcomes	Status

Progress on Transition Plan

Attach additional pages as needed and additional outcomes if developed.

Connecticut Birth to Three Form 3-1 (Revised 7/1/06)

Appendix L. *continues*

195

Section R-2 Individualized Family Service Plan (IFSP) Review: Services and Supports

Child's Name: _____ DOB: _____ Date of IFSP being reviewed: _____ Review Date: _____

Result of Review: _____

SUMMARY OF REVISED EARLY INTERVENTION SERVICES AND SUPPORTS
(To be completed after review of outcomes)

*What is going to happen (including assistive technology)	*Delivered by: (Discipline responsible)	*Location	*How Often	*How Long	*Start Date	*End Date
		code				

☐ Check here if additional pages are attached to list or clarify the services being provided or the schedule of services.

Primary service location codes: 1=home 2=setting designed for typical children 3=hospital (inpatient) 4=residential facility 5=service provider office 6=setting designed for children with delays 7=other

☐ *Check if any early intervention service cannot be achieved satisfactorily in a natural environment and attach a justification for each service.

Services are paid for by the Birth to Three System unless otherwise indicated:

Service Coordinator/Program/Discipline/phone#:

Service Coordination is provided to all families at least monthly and is most often part of the early intervention visit

Informed Consent by Parents. Check and sign below:

1. _____ I understand my rights under this program and received a written copy of *Parent Rights Under IDEA Part C* **and**

2a. _____ I give permission to carry out this Individualized Family Service Plan as written. **or**

2b. _____ I do not accept this Individualized Family Service Plan as written, however I do give permission for the following services to begin:

Parent Signature _____ Date _____ Parent Signature _____ Date _____

I have reviewed the revisions made to this Individualized Family Service Plan. I confirm the appropriateness of the diagnosis(es) as stated by the diagnostic (ICD-9) code and the recommendations for the treatment services as they are written.

Physician Signature: _____

*Print Name: _____ LIC#: _____ *Date: _____

*ICD-9 Code(s) _____

*Denotes part of the electronic record

Connecticut Birth to Three Form 3-1 (Revised 7/1/06)

Confidential Document

Appendix L. *continues*

Child's Name: _____ DOB: _____ Date: _____

JUSTIFICATION FOR EARLY INTERVENTION SERVICES THAT CANNOT BE ACHIEVED SATISFACTORILY IN A NATURAL ENVIRONMENT

LOCATION OF SERVICE: _____   SERVICE: _____

1. Explain how and why the child's outcome(s) could not be met if the service were provided in the child's natural environment with supplementary supports. If the child has not made satisfactory progress towards an outcome in a natural environment, include a description of why alternative natural environments have not been selected or outcome not modified.	
2. Explain how services provided in this location will be generalized to support the child's ability to function in his or her natural environment.	
3. Describe a plan with timelines and supports necessary to allow the child's outcome(s) to be satisfactorily achieved in his or her natural environment.	

Connecticut Birth to Three Form 3-1a (Revised 1/1/06)

Appendix L. *continues*

Child's Name: _____ DOB: _____ Date: _____

ADDITIONAL PAGE
INDIVIDUALIZED FAMILY SERVICE PLAN

_____

_____

_____

_____

_____

_____

_____

_____

_____

_____

_____

_____

_____

_____

_____

_____

_____

_____

_____

_____

_____

Connecticut Birth to Three Form 3-1 (Revised 1/1/06)

Confidential Document

Appendix L. _continued_

Example of an IEP Used in Public School Settings

INDIVIDUALIZED EDUCATION PROGRAM

STUDENT'S NAME:						
DOB		**SCHOOL YEAR**		-	**GRADE**	-

IEP INITIATION/DURATION DATES	FROM		TO	

THIS IEP WILL BE IMPLEMENTED DURING THE REGULAR SCHOOL TERM UNLESS NOTED IN EXTENDED SCHOOL YEAR SERVICES.

STUDENT PROFILE – WILL INCLUDE GENERAL STATEMENTS REGARDING:

Strengths of the student:

Parental concerns:

Student Preferences and/or Interests:

Results of the most recent evaluations:

The academic, developmental, and functional needs of the student:

Other:

For the child transitioning from EI to Preschool, justify if IEP will not be implemented on the child's 3rd birthday:

Page _____ of _____

ALSDE Approved Feb. 2012

Appendix M. Example of an IEP Used in Public School Settings *continues*

INDIVIDUALIZED EDUCATION PROGRAM

STUDENT'S NAME: _____

SPECIAL INSTRUCTIONAL FACTORS

Items checked "YES" will be addressed in this IEP:

	YES	NO
• Does the student have behavior which impedes his/her learning or the learning of others?	[ ]	[ ]
• Does the student have limited English proficiency?	[ ]	[ ]
• Does the student need instruction in Braille and the use of Braille?	[ ]	[ ]
• Does the student have communication needs (deaf or hearing impaired only)?	[ ]	[ ]
• Does the student need assistive technology devices and/or services?	[ ]	[ ]
• Does the student require specially designed P.E.?	[ ]	[ ]
• Is the student working toward alternate achievement standards and participating in the *Alabama Alternate Assessment*?	[ ]	[ ]
• Are transition services addressed in this IEP with an annual goal(s)?	[ ]	[ ]

TRANSPORTATION AS A RELATED SERVICE

Student's mode of transportation:

[ ] Regular bus   [ ] Bus for special needs   [ ] Parent contract   [ ] Other: _____

Does the student require transportation as a related service?   [ ] YES   [ ] NO

If yes, check any transportation needs:

[ ]   Bus assistance: [ ] Adult support   [ ] Medical support

[ ]   Preferential seating

[ ]   Behavioral Intervention Plan

[ ]   Wheelchair lift and securement system

[ ]   Restraint system
Specify type: _____

[ ]   Other. Specify: _____

[ ]   Bus driver and support personnel are aware of the student's behavioral and/or medical concerns.

NONACADEMIC and EXTRACURRICULAR ACTIVITIES

Will the student have the opportunity to participate in nonacademic/extracurricular activities with his/her nondisabled peers?

[ ]   YES.

[ ]   YES, with supports. Describe: _____

[ ]   NO. Explanation must be provided: _____

METHOD/FREQUENCY FOR REPORTING PROGRESS OF ATTAINING GOALS TO PARENTS

Annual Goal Progress reports will be sent to parents each time report cards are issued (every _____ weeks).

Page _____ of _____

ALSDE Approved Feb. 2012

Appendix M. *continues*

INDIVIDUALIZED EDUCATION PROGRAM

STUDENT'S NAME: _____

[ ] This student is in a middle school **course of study** that will help prepare him/her for transition.
[ ] This student was invited to the IEP Team meeting.
[ ] After prior consent of the parent or student (Age 19) was obtained, other agency representatives were invited to the IEP Team meeting.

EXIT OPTIONS (Complete for students in Grades 9-12)

[ ] Alabama High School Diploma   **Anticipated Date of Exit:**   Month: _____   Year : _____
[ ] Alabama Occupational Diploma
[ ] Graduation Certificate

PROGRAM CREDIT TO BE EARNED (Complete for students in grades 9-12)							
For each course taken, indicate program credit to be earned.	ENGLISH	MATH	SCIENCE	SOCIAL STUDIES			
Alabama High School Diploma							
Alabama Occupational Diploma							
Graduation Certificate							

TRANSITION: (Beginning not later than the first IEP to be in effect when the student is 16, or earlier if appropriate, and updated annually thereafter)

Transition Assessments (Check the assessment(s) used to determine the student's measurable transition goals):

[ ] Transition Planning Assessments   [ ] Interest Inventory   [ ] Other _____

Goals for Postsecondary Transition:

Postsecondary Education/Training Goal

_____

If **Other** is selected, specify

_____

Employment/Occupation/Career Goal

_____

If **Other** is selected, specify

_____

Community/Independent Living Goal

_____

If **Other** is selected, specify

_____

Transition Services: **Based on the student's strengths, preferences, and interests, the following coordinated transition services will reasonably enable the student to meet the postsecondary goals. Consider these service areas:** Vocational Evaluations (VE), Community Experiences (CE), Personal Management (PM), Transportation (T), Employment Development (ED), Medical (M), Postsecondary Education (PE), Living Arrangements (LA), Linkages to Agencies (LTA), Advocacy/Guardianship (AG), Financial Management (FM), and if appropriate Functional Vocational Evaluation (FVE).

	Transition Strands			
	Academics/Post Secondary Education/Training	Employment/Occupations/ Careers	Personal/ Social	Daily Living
Service(s)				

Appendix M. *continues*

INDIVIDUALIZED EDUCATION PROGRAM

STUDENT'S NAME: _____

[ ] This goal is related to the student's transition services needs.

AREA: _____

PRESENT LEVEL OF ACADEMIC ACHIEVEMENT AND FUNCTIONAL PERFORMANCE:

MEASURABLE ANNUAL GOAL related to meeting the student's needs: **DATE OF MASTERY:** _____

TYPE(S) OF EVALUATION FOR ANNUAL GOAL:

[ ] Curriculum Based Assessment   [ ] Teacher/Text Test   [ ] Teacher Observation   [ ] Grades

[ ] Data Collection   [ ] State Assessment(s)   [ ] Work Samples

[ ] Other: _____   [ ] Other: _____

BENCHMARKS:

1. _____   Date of Mastery: _____
2. _____   Date of Mastery: _____
3. _____   Date of Mastery: _____
4. _____   Date of Mastery: _____

[ ] This goal is related to the student's transition services needs.

AREA: _____

PRESENT LEVEL OF ACADEMIC ACHIEVEMENT AND FUNCTIONAL PERFORMANCE:

MEASURABLE ANNUAL GOAL related to meeting the student's needs: **DATE OF MASTERY:** _____

TYPE(S) OF EVALUATION FOR ANNUAL GOAL:

[ ] Curriculum Based Assessment   [ ] Teacher/Text Test   [ ] Teacher Observation   [ ] Grades

[ ] Data Collection   [ ] State Assessment(s)   [ ] Work Samples

[ ] Other: _____   [ ] Other: _____

BENCHMARKS:

1. _____   Date of Mastery: _____
2. _____   Date of Mastery: _____
3. _____   Date of Mastery: _____
4. _____   Date of Mastery: _____

Page _____ of _____

ALSDE Approved Feb. 2012

Appendix M. *continues*

203

INDIVIDUALIZED EDUCATION PROGRAM

Student's Name: _____

SPECIAL EDUCATION AND RELATED SERVICE(S): (Special Education, Supplementary Aids and Services, Program Modifications, Accommodations Needed for Assessments, Related Services, Assistive Technology, and Support for Personnel.)

Special Education

Service(s)	Anticipated Frequency of Service(s)	Amount of time	Beginning/Ending Duration Dates	Location of Service(s)
			to	
			to	

Related Services   [ ] Needed   [ ] Not Needed

Service(s)	Anticipated Frequency of Service(s)	Amount of time	Beginning/Ending Duration Dates	Location of Service(s)
			to	
			to	

Supplementary Aids and Services   [ ] Needed   [ ] Not Needed

Service(s)	Anticipated Frequency of Service(s)	Amount of time	Beginning/Ending Duration Dates	Location of Service(s)
			to	
			to	

Program Modifications   [ ] Needed   [ ] Not Needed

Service(s)	Anticipated Frequency of Service(s)	Amount of time	Beginning/Ending Duration Dates	Location of Service(s)
			to	
			to	

Accommodations Needed for Assessments   [ ] Needed   [ ] Not Needed

Service(s)	Anticipated Frequency of Service(s)	Amount of time	Beginning/Ending Duration Dates	Location of Service(s)
			to	
			to	

Assistive Technology   [ ] Needed   [ ] Not Needed

Service(s)	Anticipated Frequency of Service(s)	Amount of time	Beginning/Ending Duration Dates	Location of Service(s)
			to	
			to	

Support for Personnel   [ ] Needed   [ ] Not Needed

Service(s)	Anticipated Frequency of Service(s)	Amount of time	Beginning/Ending Duration Dates	Location of Service(s)
			to	
			to	

Page _____ of _____

ALSDE Approved Feb. 2012

Appendix M. *continues*

INDIVIDUALIZED EDUCATION PROGRAM

STUDENT'S NAME: _____

TRANSFER OF RIGHTS

(Beginning not later than the IEP that will be in effect when the student reaches 18 years of age.)

Date student was informed that the rights under the IDEA will transfer to him/her at the age of 19 _____

The IEP Team has considered the need for extended school year services.   [ ] Yes   [ ] No

LEAST RESTRICTIVE ENVIRONMENT

Does this student attend the school (or for a preschool-age student, participate in the environment) he/she would attend if nondisabled?   [ ] Yes   [ ] No
If no, explain:

_____

Does this student receive all special education services with nondisabled peers? [ ] Yes [ ] No
If no, explain (explanation may not be solely because of needed modifications in the general curriculum):

_____

| [ ] 6-21 YEARS OF AGE | [ ] 3-5 YEARS OF AGE |

Least Restricted Environment:

_____

## COPY OF IEP	## COPY OF *SPECIAL EDUCATION RIGHTS*
Was a copy of the IEP given to parent/student (age 19) at the IEP Team meeting? [ ] Yes [ ] No	Was a copy of the *Special Education Rights* given to parent/student (age 19) at the IEP Team meeting? [ ] Yes [ ] No
If no, date sent: _____	If no, date sent: _____

Date copy of **amended** IEP provided/sent to parent/student (age 19) _____

THE FOLLOWING PEOPLE ATTENDED AND PARTICIPATED IN THE MEETING TO DEVELOP THIS IEP.

Position	Signature	Date
Parent		
Parent		
General Education Teacher		
Special Education Teacher		
LEA Representative		
Someone Who Can Interpret The Instructional Implications Of The Evaluation Results		
Student		
Career/Technical Education Representative		
Other Agency Representative		

INFORMATION FROM PEOPLE NOT IN ATTENDANCE

Position	Name	Date

Page ____ of _____

ALSDE Approved Feb. 2012

Appendix M. *continued*

Example of an Annual Goal Progress Report Form Used in Public Schools

Annual Goal Progress Report

Student Name: _____

Student ID Number: _____

Date Sent: _____

IEP Initiation/Duration Dates From: _____ to _____

School Year: _____

IEP Annual Review Date: _____

Use the legends below to evaluate the student's progress toward the annual goals. The 1st column should indicate the *Report of Progress* using the numbers 1-4. The 2nd column should indicate the *Extent of Progress* using the numbers 1-4.

Report of Progress on Annual Goals

1. Goal has been met.
2. Some progress made.
3. Very little progress made.
4. No progress made.

Extent of Progress Toward Meeting the Annual Goals

1. Goal mastered.
2. Anticipate mastery.
3. Do not anticipate mastery.
4. *NA* Not applicable during this grading period.

Report/Extent of Progress														
Record Date of Reporting Periods														

Measurable Annual Goals

School System
School Name

Appendix N. Example of an Annual Goal Progress Report Form Used in Public Schools *continues*

6/1/2006

Annual Goal Progress Report

Student Name _____   Student ID Number: _____

Reporting Periods	Comments

Special Education Teacher/
Case Manager Name: _____   Telephone Number: _____

Parent/Guardian Signature: _____   Date Signed: _____

*** Hard copy should be placed in student's special education record. ***

(School System)
(School Name)

6/1/2006

Appendix N. continued

Examples of University Clinic Long-Term Treatment Reports

NAME: John Gates

AGE: 15

ADDRESS: 1234 Oak St.
           Anytown, USA

DATE OF REPORT: 5-1-12

CLINICIAN: K. Gates

FILE NUMBER: 00-345-2

D.O.B.: 1-20-07

PHONE NUMBER: 334-123-4567

PERIOD COVERED: Spring 2012

Current Background Information

John is a 15-year-old male who has a history of stuttering since early childhood. He will be entering the tenth grade this fall in a regular education classroom. According to his parents, John is a "very good student" and is involved with several sports teams at his school. He was initially evaluated at this clinic on October 1, 2011. According to the *Stuttering Severity Instrument (SSI-3),* he exhibits a moderate to severe fluency disorder which has a significant impact on his daily interactions. John is receiving speech therapy through the public schools in a group setting once a week for 30 minutes. He was referred to this clinic for additional assessment and individual treatment.

Current Evaluation Results

Date of Evaluation: October 1, 2011

Assessment Tool: *Stuttering Severity Instrument (SSI-4)*

Scores are as follows:

    Frequency: 12

    Duration: 10

    Physical Concomitants: 10

    Total Score: 32

    Percentile rank: 75–80%

    Severity rating: Moderate–Severe

Assessment Tool: *Overall Assessment of the Speaker's Experience of Stuttering* (OASES)

    Section I: General Information Impact Score: 3.3 (Mod.-Severe)

    Section II: Your Reactions to Stuttering Impact Score: 4.0 (Severe)

    Section III: Communication in Daily Situations Impact Score: 3.4 (Mod.-Severe)

    Section IV: Quality of Life Impact Score: 3.0 (Mod.-Severe)

    Total Impact Score: 61 (Moderate to Severe)

Reports most difficulty with talking on the phone, speaking with unfamiliar people and class presentations.

LTG 1: The client will achieve a comfortable level of fluency at the conversational level in social and academic settings.

STO A: The client will utilize a smooth, controlled rate during structured reading tasks with 80% accuracy.

Baseline Data:	2-7-12	3/12 = 25%
Final Data	2-28-12	11/15 = 73%

Materials: Eight to ten word sentences from *HELP* workbook

Cues: Clinician models smooth rate; "Remember to smooth out your speech"

Reinforcement: Verbal praise, replay audiotape

John made significant progress during structured reading tasks. He stated that it was easier to use a controlled rate while reading, because he "gets into a rhythm."

STO B: The client will utilize smooth and easy speech during structured conversation in order to decrease disfluencies to less than 10% during a 60-minute session.

Baseline Data:	2-28-12	31% disfluent
Final Data:	4-18-12	18% disfluent

Materials: *Life Stories* cards, *Converstation* game, spontaneous conversation with clinician

Cues: Verbal cue (remember to keep your voice turned on)

Reinforcement: Verbal praise, "I like how you said that," "Very smooth speech."

Overall, John's percentage of disfluencies decreased over the course of the semester, although it fluctuated significantly. John stated that when he was under a lot of stress due to schoolwork and responsibilities with sports, he felt it was more difficult to maintain fluent speech.

STO C: The client will utilize the *Easy Onset* technique during a structured reading task with 90% accuracy.

Baseline Data:	3-14-12	10% accuracy
Final Data:	3-28-12	80% accuracy

Materials: Short paragraphs from *The Source for Apraxia Therapy* workbook, newspaper and magazine articles.

Cues: "Remember to prolong the first sound in the word."
    Clinician models technique

Reinforcement: Replay videotape, verbal praise

John did well using Easy Onset, although he stated that he wasn't really comfortable doing it, and that most likely, he won't use this technique outside of the therapy room; therefore, it will not be targeted in future sessions.

continues

STO D: The client will utilize the *Easy Onset* technique when having difficulty initiating spontaneous speech on 4/5 communication opportunities.

Baseline Data: 3-28-12   0 times
Final Data   4-18-12   4/10 times

Materials: None

Cues: "It sounded like you had difficulty with the word _____." "Let's try that again."
      Clinician models technique

Reinforcement: Verbal praise

As stated above, John reports that although he is able to have success using Easy Onset, he is not very comfortable using it.

Summary/Recommendations

John made significant progress this semester regarding his awareness of moments of disfluency, as well as identifying which strategies were most helpful for him. Even though he initially reported that his stuttering does not hold him back in any way, he eventually shared with the clinician that he sometimes avoids certain speaking situations such as phone conversations and oral presentations. With increased confidence regarding use of his techniques, John has a more positive attitude regarding his speech, and stated that he felt therapy had been very helpful for him. It is recommended that John continue with speech therapy at the A.U. Speech and Hearing Clinic at a frequency of 1 time per week for 60-minute sessions during the fall semester. Treatment goals should focus on:

1. Increased awareness of moments of stuttering and avoidance techniques within the therapy setting.
2. Increasing efficiency in using fluency shaping techniques, (easy onset, smooth transitions between words and phrases).
3. Improving fluency in unstructured speaking situations.
4. Increase self-monitoring outside of the therapy setting.

TREATMENT REPORT

NAME: Michael Spears

AGE: 4.8 years

D.O.B.: 4/12/07

ADDRESS: 123 Main St.
         Auburn, AL 36830

TEL. NUMBER: 334- 844-9600

FILE NUMBER: 00-11-22

PARENT'S NAME: Steve & Mary Spears

DIAGNOSIS: Articulation/Language

DATE OF REPORT: December 2012

PERIOD COVERED: Fall 2012

CLINICIAN: Jane Smith

NUMBER SESSIONS ATTENDED: <u>18</u> OUT OF <u>22</u> SCHEDULED SESSIONS

SCHEDULED SESSIONS: <u>30</u> MINUTES <u>2</u> TIMES PER WEEK

Current Background Information

Michael is a 4.8-year-old male who has been receiving services from Auburn University Speech and Hearing Clinic (AUSHC) since spring semester of 2012 for an articulation and language delay. During the evaluation, Mrs. Spears reported that Michael was the product of a full-term unremarkable pregnancy and delivery. Michael has a history of frequent colds and ear infections and underwent tonsillectomy and bilateral PE tube placement in March, 2011. He attends a preschool classroom three mornings a week at Jacob's Ladder and will be entering kindergarten next in the fall of 2013. He currently receives no other speech/language services.

Current Evaluation Results

Date of evaluation: 01/16/12

Assessment tool: Language Sample

Results: An informal language sample was obtained through play. Michael exhibited an MLU of 2.5 during the assessment. His pragmatics, play skills and social interaction were judged to be within normal limits. Michael consistently understands and uses prepositions and descriptive concepts. Michael displayed appropriate attention and frequently imitated the clinician using 3+word utterances. Results of the assessment indicate that increasing MLU as well as knowledge and use of age-appropriate linguistic and grammatical concepts should be targeted. Michael appeared to be functioning at an age-appropriate level with respect to all other skills.

Date of Evaluation: 01/16/12

Assessment tool: *Goldman-Fristoe Test of Articulation-2nd Edition* (GFTA-2)

Results:

    Raw Score: 24

    Standard Score: 91 (27th percentile)

    Age-Equivalent: 3.4

Michael exhibits some developmental speech sound errors, such as w/r, w/l, and d/z; however, he also exhibits errors regarding sounds he should have mastered (k, g) for his age. He was stimulable for correct production of /g/ with phonetic and tactile cues at the word level.

continues

215

Appendix O. *continued*

Date of Evaluation: 01/16/12

Assessment tool: *Pre-school Language Scale-5th Edition* (PLS-5)

Results:

    Scores: Receptive Language:
                  Standard Score: 87 (19th percentile)
                  Age-Equivalent: 3.9

                  Expressive Language:
                  Standard Score: 84 (14th percentile)
                  Age-Equivalent: 3.10

                  Total Language:
                  Standard Score: 84 (14th percentile)
                  Age-Equivalent: 3.11

Standard scores between 85 and 115 are considered within normal limits; therefore, Michael exhibits a mild expressive language delay and low average receptive abilities when compared to his same age peers. Michael had difficulty with several age-appropriate linguistic concepts, such as negation, possessive pronouns, telling how an object is used, and answering questions about hypothetical events.

Objectives & Progress

LTG I: The client will improve production of all age-appropriate phonemes in order increase overall intelligibility at the conversational level.

STO A: The client will produce /g/ initial at the imitative word level while playing a game with 90% accuracy.

            Baseline Data: date: 08/29/12   results: 5/10 = 75%
                                                               Cue 1: 2/10 = 20%
                                                                 Cue 2: 1/10 = 10%

            Final Semester Data: date: 09/28/12   results: 9/10 = 90%
                                                              Cue 1: 1/10 = 10%

Target: go, goat, gum, game, golf, ghost, gate (one syllable /g/ initial words)

Materials: Webber articulation cards, Fish-n-Say, Bingo

Cues: 1. Verbal cue "Remember your back sound."
                  2. Phonemic cue
                  3. Tactile cue

Effective Cue: Phonemic cue

Reinforcers: Conditioned generalized reinforcement, Primary reinforcement (goldfish)

Michael consistently substitutes /d/ for /g/ in all positions in spontaneous speech. This semester, he made significant progress within the first month of therapy and was able to advance to the spontaneous word level after meeting criteria at the imitative level. Michael enjoyed earning stickers for each trial to trade in for a prize at the end of the session.

STO B: The client will produce /g/ initial at the spontaneous word level while naming pictures with 90% accuracy.

	Baseline Data:	date: 09/28/12	results: 5/10 = 50%
			Cue 2: 1/10 = 10%
			Cue 3: 2/10 = 20%
	Final Semester Data:	date: 11/28/12	results: 7/10 = 70%
			Cue 2: 2/10 = 20%

Target: golf, ghost, gate, gorilla, game, goat (one syllable /g/ initial words)

Materials: Worksheets, home-made articulation cards

Cues: 1. Verbal cue, "Remember your back sound."
                 2. Phonemic cue
                 3. Full model

Effective Cues: Phonemic cue

Reinforcers: Verbal praise "Good /g/ sound"
                 Stickers

This objective was targeted initially at mid-semester after Michael met the goal for imitative words. He met criteria for the objective during the last 3 sessions and it is recommended that Michael advance to the imitative phrase level when he returns to therapy.

STO C: The client will imitatively produce /k/ initial in CV and CVC words with 90% accuracy.

	Baseline Data:	date: 09/28/07	results: 5/10 = 50%
			Cue 2: 1/10 = 10%
			Cue 3: 2/10 = 20%
	Final Semester Data:	date: 11/28/07	results: 6/10 = 60%
			Cue 2: 1/10 = 10%
			Cue 3: 2/10 = 20%

Target: key, cow, kick, cat, cot, kiss, can, cup (one syllable /k/ initial words, CV combinations)

Materials: Worksheets, home-made articulation cards

Cues: 1. Verbal cue, "Remember your back sound."
                 2. Phonemic cue
                 3. Full model

Effective Cues: Full model

Reinforcers: Verbal praise "Good /k/ sound"
                 Stickers

Progress with this goal has been limited and variable. Although he has mastered /k/ at the imitative syllable level, he is having difficulty with consistently producing it in simple CV words. During the last month of therapy, performance varied between 30 and 70%. However, Michael is exhibiting increased self-awareness for errors and is frequently self-correcting prior to cueing.

continues

LTG II: The client will improve receptive and expressive language skills to an age-appropriate level.

STO A: The client will correctly use possessive pronouns during a structured language activity utilizing visual cues with 90% accuracy.

Baseline Data:	date: 08/28/12	results:	4/10 = 40%
			Cue 2: 6/10 = 60%
Final Semester Data:	date: 11/28/12	results:	9/10 = 90%
			Cue 1: 1/10 = 10%

Target: Possessive pronouns (his, hers, mine)

Materials: Webber cards, language/grammar games

Cues: 1. Repeat stimulus
                   2. Choice cue
                   3. Full model

Effective Cues: Repetition of stimulus

Reinforcers: Verbal praise (Nice work!)
                 Basketball

Michael made consistent progress with comprehension and use of possessive pronouns, and met criteria during the last 2 sessions. Initially, he performed better when given a choice cue, but by the end of the semester, he only required the stimulus to be repeated. Michael was motivated by being allowed to shoot the basketball after working for 10 minutes.

STO B: The client will increase spontaneous MLU to 4.0 during structured play activities with the clinician.

Baseline Data:	date: 09/09/12	results: 3.0
Final Semester Data:	date: 11/28/12	results: 4.0

Target: Semantic relations: object + action; agent + action; recurrence + action; location + object

Materials: A variety of toys including the farm, cars, telephone

Cues: 1. Giving choices
                   2. Model utterances emphasizing word production

Effective Cues: Choices

Reinforcers: Verbal praise, "I like how you said that," "I heard you say, I want the blue car."
                 Stickers

A variety of materials were used to target this goal. Michael was observed to use the longest and most variety of utterances when the farm, cars, and blocks were involved. Michael's increase in utterances includes comments about objects, actions, and imperatives. Michael has met this goal and is using an age appropriate MLU at this time.

STO C: The client will demonstrate knowledge of the concept of negation by pointing to the correct picture from a field of four (4) with 75% accuracy following an auditory stimulus from the clinician.

Target: Increase knowledge of negation (which one is not crying, which nest has no eggs)

Materials: Various picture cards

Cues:
1. Repeat stimulus
2. Emphasize "not" and eliminate one choice
3. Give him 2 choices only

Summary

Michael made consistent progress throughout the semester and he met several of his goals. He is now functioning at an age appropriate level with regard to expressive and receptive language. Michael was attentive at the beginning of most sessions, but after 15–20 minutes, he became easily distracted, and required redirection. Michael was motivated to participate in articulation tasks when they were structured as drill/play and followed by reinforcement such as shooting the basketball. A consistent set of stimuli was used for all targeted articulation goals. Mr. and Mrs. Spears were given a home program after the first treatment session, and worked with Michael twice weekly to target articulation and language. Therapy next semester should continue to focus on correct production of /k/ and /g/ in all word positions.

Recommendations

It is recommended that Michael enroll in treatment at the Auburn University Speech & Hearing Clinic at a frequency of 2 times per week for 30-minute sessions. Treatment goals should focus on:

1. Improving production of /g/ initial, medial and final in words and phrases
2. Improving production of /k/ initial at the spontaneous word level
3. Improving production of /k/ initial at the imitative phrase level
4. Continue to monitor language production and acquisition of pre-academic skills

_____   _____
Jane Smith, B.S.   Amanda Clark, M.S., CCC/SLP
Graduate Clinician   Clinical Supervisor/SLP

cc:
Steve & Mary Spears
Ms. Sparks, CCC-SLP; Auburn School System

APPENDIX P

Writing Measurable Goals and Objectives

WRITING MEASURABLE GOALS AND OBJECTIVES

LEARNER PERFORMANCE	QUALITY	CRITERIA	CONDITIONS

• Alphabetize
• Answer
• Arrange
• Ask
• Bring
• Chart
• Choose
• Compare
• Compile
• Complete
• Compose
• Contrast
• Contribute
• Correct count
• Create
• Decode
• Define
• Demonstrate
• Describe
• Determine
• Differentiate
• Discriminate
• Does not ___
• Edit
• Explain
• Follow
• Generate
• Give
• Greet
	• Identify
	• Include
	• Initiate
	• Imitate
	• Label
	• List
	• Maintain
	• Make
	• Match
	• Name
	• Organize
	• Outline
	• Paraphrase
	• Point
	• Pronounce
	• Provide
	• Read
	• Record
	• Retell
	• Say
	• Select
	• Self correct
	• Share
	• Solve
	• Speak
	• Spell
	• Summarize
	• Type
	• Volunteer
		• Independently
		• With prompting
		  – Verbal
		  – Visual
		  – Physical
		  – Gestural
		  – Limited
		• In the correct order
		• With correct capitalization
		• With correct punctuation of periods, questions marks, commas…
		• With a main idea and (#) of supporting details
		• Legibly
		• Without assistance
		• With minimal assistance
		• Instantly and correctly
		• On the first attempt
		• At a level judged satisfactory by teacher
		• With no more than one redirection
		• With a score of ___ from the ___ grade writing rubric
			Frequency
			• ___ x each day
			• ___ x in ___ minutes each day
			• ___ consecutive days
			• Fewer than ___ minutes each week
			• Whenever it appears
			Duration
			• For ___ minutes
			• For ___ repetitions in ___ (amount of time)
			Accuracy
			• ___ % of the time
			• ___ our of ___ trials
			• No more than ___ errors
			• With ___ errors
			• No more than random error (define)
			Latency/Speed
			• ___ words per minute
			• ___ letters per minute
			• In less than ___ minute
			• ___ seconds or less
			• Complete work in ___ minutes
			• Within ___ minutes of a verbal prompt
			Intensity
			With ___ pounds of pressure/force
				Location
				• During lunch
				• In a large group
				• In a small group
				• In a 1:1 setting
				• During free/play time
				• Across environments
				• During time readings
				• In a sharing routine
				• In the community
				Givens
				• Given ___ paragraphs
				• Given pictures
				• Given unfamiliar material
				• Given words or letters
				• Given a topic
				• Given a story starter
				• Given CVC words
				• Given a calculator
				• Given a model
				• Given a writing prompt
				Misc
				• With typical peers
				• With adults
				• With ___ software (do not use brand names)
				• With ___ grade vocabulary
				• With two hands
				• With L/R hand
				• With a (#) key hit sequence through use of ___ (AT)
				• Through use of ___ strategy/behavior
				• In (type of) writing
				• In (grade level) test/material

NON-MEASURABLE: comprehend, Enjoy, feel, increase (from what to what?), know listen, learn, manipulate (how?), participate (how?), realize. understand

Adapted from HCESC Smart Sheet, Chalfant and McGraw, 4/2004

Appendix P. Writing Measurable Goals and Objectives

Example of a Long-Term Care Facility Progress Report

ST - Therapist Progress Report

Date :

PATIENT		ID		PAYOR	
PHYSICIAN		MED DX			
TREATMENT DX1			TREATMENT DX2		
START OF CARE		END OF CARE		MED DX ONSET	

Number of Skilled Treatments: ____ since last report

Number of Missed Treatments: ____

Reason for Missed Treatments:

Goal Name	Goal	Prior Level of Function	Current Level of Function	Goal Date

Patient continues to require skilled PT services to focus on:

Analysis of Functional Outcome / Clinical Impression:

Skilled Services Provided since Last Report:

Patient / Caregiver Training:

Remaining Functional Deficits / Underlying Impairments:

Impact on Burden of Care / Daily Life:

Updates to Treatment Approach:

Precautions:

Prognosis for Futher Progress:

Signed by Therapist: _____   Date: _____

Facility Name: _____   Page: _____

Appendix Q. Example of a Long-Term Care Facility Progress Report

APPENDIX R

Examples of Data Sheets

DOCUMENTATION FORM

Client: _____ **Clinician:** _____

FILE # _____ **Short-term objective:** _____

DATE _____

PROCEDURE, MATERIALS, REINFORCERS

Trials-Record C or Cue # for each trial

C- Correct	Cue 1	Cue 2	Cue 3
/	/	/	/
%	%	%	%

DATE _____

PROCEDURE, MATERIALS, REINFORCERS

Trials-Record C or Cue # for each trial

C –Correct	Cue 1	Cue 2	Cue 3
/	/	/	/
%	%	%	%

DATE _____

PROCEDURE, MATERIALS, REINFORCERS

Trials-Record C or Cue # for each trial

C – Correct	Cue 1	Cue 2	Cue 3
/	/	/	/
%	%	%	%

DATE _____

PROCEDURE, MATERIALS, REINFORCERS

Trials-Record C or Cue # for each trial

C- Correct	Cue 1	Cue 2	Cue 3
/	/	/	/
%	%	%	%

DATE _____

PROCEDURE, MATERIALS, REINFORCERS

Trials-Record C or Cue # for each trial

C- Correct	Cue 1	Cue 2	Cue3
/	/	/	/
%	%	%	%

DATE _____

PROCEDURE, MATERIALS, REINFORCERS

Trials-Record C or Cue # for each trial

C- Correct	Cue 1	Cue 2	Cue 3
/	/	/	/
%	%	%	%

Appendix R. Examples of Data Sheets *continues*

Early Language Data Sheet

Date:	Client name:		Clinician:
	S=spontaneous G=gesture/sign	PA=physical assistance	I-imitative
Greeting Eye Contact			
Joint Attention			
Commenting			
Requesting			
Protesting			
Answering "WH" and Yes/no questions			

Appendix R. *continues*

OBJECTIVE/ACTIVITY

CUEING HIERARCHY

DATA (NUMBER & PERCENTAGE)

1._____
_____
_____
_____
_____
_____
_____

CUEING HIERARCHY	DATA (NUMBER & PERCENTAGE)
NO CUES	

2._____
_____
_____
_____
_____
_____
_____

CUEING HIERARCHY	DATA (NUMBER & PERCENTAGE)
NO CUES	

3._____
_____
_____
_____
_____
_____
_____

CUEING HIERARCHY	DATA (NUMBER & PERCENTAGE)
NO CUES	

Appendix R. *continued*

Examples of SOAP Notes

SOAP Note

Client: Louise Jackson   Date: 9/22/12
File #: Holding   Clinician: L. Willis

SUBJECT	Mrs. Jackson arrived on time with her husband. She was compliant throughout the session and appeared to exert maximum effort during all activities. She engaged in simple conversation with the clinician by using single words and neologisms and occasional gestures to communicate. Assessment was continued to establish meaningful goals for future sessions.

OBJECTIVE	1. Functional object use with 90% accuracy:
	   10/10 = 100%
	2. Spontaneous simple sentence completion with 60% accuracy with minimal cueing:
	   1/12 = 8% with phonemic cue
	   10/12 = 83% with full model
	   1/12 = 8% with written cue and full model
	3. Spontaneous common object naming with 60% accuracy:
	   2/10 = 20%
	   1/10 = 10% with semantic cues
	   3/10 = 30% with phonemic cues
	
	   She was unable to imitate "toothbrush" or "paintbrush" despite full model.
	4. Match written word to picture from field of 3 with 90% accuracy: 6/6 = 100%
	5. Match written phrase to picture from field of 3 with 90% accuracy: 10/12 = 83%
	6. Simple general yes/no questions with 90% accuracy: 20/20

ASSESSMENT	Mrs. Jackson frequently attempted to vocalize during the session with vocal approximations, neologisms, and paraphasias. Rarely was she able to meaningfully use a true word during unstructured interaction. Her expressive strengths include imitation of the clinician at the single word/phrase level and oral reading. She appeared to understand some simple conversation with cues but had difficulty when an AAC device was discussed. Her husband offered suggestions of items to be included in a trial AAC book. Mrs. Jackson again exceeded criteria for the reading and auditory comprehension tasks.
PLAN	-Increase cues for simple sentence completion task. -Create simple AAC device for trial use at home. -Increase difficulty for reading comprehension to simple sentences. -Increase difficulty of auditory questions to moderate level. -Target receptive ability of following 1–2 step commands. -Discharge goal for functional object use due to exceeding criteria for three consecutive sessions.

Appendix S. Examples of SOAP Notes *continues*

SOAP Note

Client: <u>Charlie Dunn</u>   Date: <u>10/15/12</u>

File #: <u>00-65-98</u>   Clinician: <u>J. Dozen</u>

SUBJECTIVE	Charlie was tired today. Ms. Dunn reported that he had missed his morning nap. She also noted that he "did real well with his home program" this week.
OBJECTIVE	The client will produce /k/ initial at the spontaneous word level while naming picture cards with 90% accuracy. 7/10 = 70% Cue 1: 2/10 = 20% Cue 2: 1/10 = 10% The client will spontaneously name pictures depicting common verbs during joint book reading with the clinician with 90% accuracy. 5/10 = 50% Cue 2: 2/10 = 20% Cue 3: 1/10 = 10% The client will spontaneously produce a minimum of ten 4-5 word sentences during 10 minutes of picture description. Spontaneous: 3 Cue 1: 6 Cue 2: 8
ASSESSMENT	Charlie continues to use /t/ for /k/ at times; however, he is requiring less cues for placement than in previous sessions. A new book was used to address verbs today and accuracy was subsequently decreased. Charlie enjoyed the pictures during the sentence objective since they were related to baseball. He did require significant cueing to include articles.
PLAN	Due to not meeting criteria, all of the above objectives should be targeted next session, with verbal praise and stickers as reinforcement. Use the same stimuli for objectives 2 and 3 to determine if accuracy will be increased. Vary picture cards for /k/ to assess generalization.

Appendix S. *continued*

Examples of Long-Term Graphs

Appendix T. Examples of Long-Term Graphs

References

Alabama State Department of Education. (n.d.). *Mastering the maze*. Retrieved May 2, 2012, from http://www.alsde.edu.

American Academy of Pediatrics. (2007). Professionalism in pediatrics. *Pediatrics, 120*(4), 895–897.

American Speech-Language Hearing Association, ASHA Committee on Supervision. (1985). Clinical supervision in speech-language pathology. *ASHA, 27*, 57–60.

American Speech-Language-Hearing Association (ASHA). (2003). ASHA code of ethics. Retrieved April 26, 2012, from http://www.asha.org/docs/html/ET2010-00309.html

American Speech-Language-Hearing Association (ASHA). (2004). Evidence-based practice (EBP). Retrieved May 2, 2012, from http://www.asha.org/members/ebp/default

American Speech-Language-Hearing Association (ASHA). (2005). Issues in ethics statement: Cultural competence. Retrieved May 3, 2012, from http://www.asha.org/docs/html/PI2011-00326.html

American Speech-Language Hearing Association (ASHA). (2007). *Scope of practice in speech-language pathology*. Rockville, MD: Author.

Anderson, J. (1988). *The supervisory process in speech-language pathology and audiology*. Austin, TX: Pro-Ed.

Atkins, C. P. (2007). Graduate SLP/Aud clinicians on counseling: Self-perceptions and awareness of boundaries. *Contemporary Issues in Communication Science and Disorders, 34*, 4–11.

Battle, D. (1997). Multicultural considerations in counseling communicatively disordered persons and their families. In T. Crowe (Ed.), *Applications of counseling in speech-language pathology and audiology* (pp. 118–144). Baltimore, MD: Williams & Wilkins.

Battle, D. (2002). *Communication disorders in multicultural populations*. Boston, MA: Butterworth-Heinemann.

Boone, D., McFarlane, S., Von Berg, S., & Zraick, R. (2010). *The voice and voice therapy*. Needham Heights, MA: Allyn & Bacon.

Brehm, B., Breen, P., Brown, B., Long, L., Smith, R., Wall, A., & Warren, N. S. (2006). An interdisciplinary approach to introducing professionalism. *American Journal of Pharmaceutical Education, 70*(4), 1–5, Article 81.

Brown, R. (1973). *A first language: The early stages*. Boston, MA: Harvard University Press.

Capuzzi, D., & Gross, D. (2003). *Counseling and psychotherapy*. Columbus, OH: Merrill.

Centers for Medicare and Medicaid Services (CMS). Retrieved May 15, 2012, from http://www.cms.hhs.gov

Clooman, P., Davis, F., & Burnett, C. (1999). Interdisciplinary education in clinical ethics: A work in progress. *Holistic Nursing Practice, 13*, 9–12.

Consumer Driven Health Care. (n.d.). *Glossary definition of third party payment*. Retrieved May 2, 2012, from http://cdhc.ncpa.org

Council for Exceptional Children (CEC). Retrieved June 1, 2012, from http://www.cec.sped.org

Crowe, T. (1997). *Applications of counseling in speech-language pathology and audiology*. Baltimore, MD: Williams & Wilkins.

Damico, J. (1987). Addressing language concerns in the schools: The SLP as consultant. *Journal of Childhood Communication Disorders, 11*, 17–40.

Emerick, L. (1969). *The parent interview*. Danville, IL: Interstate.

Family Educational Rights and Privacy Act (FERPA). Retrieved June 1, 2012, from http://www.ed.gov/policy/gen/guid/fpco/ferpa/index.html

Ferguson, M. (1991). Collaborative/consultative service delivery: An introduction. *Language, Speech, and Hearing Services in Schools, 22*, 147.

Fourie, R. J. (2009). Qualitative study of the therapeutic relationship in speech and language therapy: Perspectives of adults with acquired communication and swallowing disorders. *International Journal of Language and Communication Disorders, 44*(6), 979–999.

Fourie, R. J. (2011). *Therapeutic processes for communication disorders: A guide for clinicians.* New York, NY: Psychology Press.

Frassinelli, L., Superior, K., & Meyers, J. (1983). A consultation model for speech and language intervention. *Journal of the American Speech-Language-Hearing Association, 25*(11), 25–30.

French, S., & Sim, J. (1993). *Writing: A guide for therapists.* Oxford, UK: Butterworth-Heinemann.

Frymark, T. (2003, May 27). FIM or foe? Functional independence measures fall short, data show. *ASHA Leader.*

Fujiki, M., & Brinton, B. (1984). Supplementing language therapy: Working with the classroom teachers. *Language, Speech, and Hearing Services in Schools, 15,* 98–109.

Gottwald, S., & Parris, D. (2006, November). *Helping people change: Teaching counseling skills in clinical practicum.* Presented at the national convention of the American Speech-Language-Hearing Association, Miami, FL.

Gregory, H. (2002). *Stuttering therapy: Rationale and procedures.* Needham Heights, MA: Allyn & Bacon.

Hackney, H., & Cormier, S. (1994). *Counseling strategies and interventions* (4th ed.). Boston, MA: Allyn & Bacon.

Hammer, D., Berger, B., & Beardsley, R. (2003). Student professionalism. *American Journal of Pharmaceutical Education, 67,* 1–29.

Haynes, W., & Hartman, D. (1975). The agony of report writing: A new look at an old problem. *Journal of the National Student Speech and Hearing Association, 3,* 7–15.

Haynes, W., & Johnson, C. (2009). *Understanding research and evidence-based practice in communication disorders: A primer for students and practitioners.* Boston, MA: Allyn & Bacon.

Haynes, W., Moran, M., & Pindzola, R. (2006). *Communication disorders in the classroom* (4th ed.). Boston, MA: Jones & Bartlett.

Haynes, W., & Oratio, A. R. (1978). A study of clients' perceptions of therapeutic effectiveness. *Journal of Speech and Hearing Disorders, 43,* 21–33.

Haynes, W., & Pindzola, R. (2008). *Diagnosis and evaluation in speech pathology* (7th ed.). Boston, MA: Allyn & Bacon.

Haynes, W., & Pindzola, R. (2012). *Diagnosis and evaluation in speech pathology* (8th ed.). Upper Saddle River, NJ: Pearson.

Health Information Portability and Accountability Act (HIPAA). Retrieved July 8, 2008, from http://www.hhs.gov/ocr/hipaa/

Hegde, M., & Davis, D. (1995). *Clinical methods and practicum in speech-language pathology* (2nd ed.). San Diego, CA: Singular.

Horton-Ikard, R., & Munoz, M. (2010). Addressing multicultural issues in communication sciences and disorders. *Contemporary Issues in Communication Sciences and Disorders, 37,* 167–173.

Individuals with Disabilities Education Act. (IDEA, 2004). (IDEA Part C and Related Topics). Retrieved October 15, 2007, from http://www.ideapartnership.org/topicdetail.cfm?topicid=33

Johnson, C. E. (2012). *Auditory rehabilitation: A contemporary issues approach.* Boston, MA: Pearson.

Kaderavek, J. N., Laux, J. M., & Mills, N. H. (2004). A counseling training module for students in speech-language pathology training programs. *Contemporary Issues in Communication Sciences and Disorders, 31,* 153–161.

Kahmi, A., Vanleer, E., Lundgren, K. Verdolini, K., & Bernstein-Ratner, N. (2009, November). *EBP: The promise and the reality.* Presented at the national convention of the American Speech-Language-Hearing Association, New Orleans, LA.

Klein, H., & Moses, N. (1999). *Intervention planning for children with communication disorders: A guide for clinical practicum and professional practice.* Boston, MA: Allyn & Bacon.

Knepflar, K. (1976). Report writing for private practitioners. In R. Battin & D. Fox (Eds.), *Private practice in audiology and speech pathology* (pp. 115–136). New York, NY: Grune and Stratton.

Lemke, A., & Dublinske, S. (2008). Achieving excellence in member service: ASHA's strategic pathway. *ASHA Leader, 13*(1), 20–21.

Locke, J. L. (1980). The inference of speech perception in the phonologically disordered child. Part I. A rationale, some criteria, the conventional tests. *Journal of Speech and Hearing Disorders, 40,* 431–444.

Magnotta, O. (1991). Looking beyond tradition. *Language, Speech, and Hearing Services in Schools, 22,* 150–151.

Luterman, D. M. (2001). *Counseling persons with communication disorders and their families* (4th ed.). Austin, TX: Pro-Ed.

Margolis, R. H. (2004, August 3). Boosting memory with informational counseling: Helping patients understand the nature of disorders and how to manage them. *ASHA Leader.*

Marvin, C. (1987). Consultation services: Changing roles for SLPs. *Journal of Childhood Communication Disorders, 11*(1), 1–16.

Matarazzo, J., & Wiens, A. (1972). *The interview: Research on its anatomy and structure.* Chicago, IL: Aldine-Atherton.

McQuire, M., & Lorch, S. (1968). A model for the study of dyadic communication. *Journal of Nervous and Mental Disease, 146,* 221–229.

Mehrabian, A. (1972). *Nonverbal communication.* Chicago, IL: Aldine Atherton.

Meitus, I. (1991). Clinical report and letter writing. In I. Meitus & B. Weinberg (Eds.), *Diagnosis in speech-language pathology* (pp. 287–307). Boston, MA: Allyn & Bacon.

Middleton, G., Pannbacker, M., Vekovius, G. T., Sanders, K. L., & Pluett, V. (2001). *Report writing for speech-language pathologists.* Upper Saddle River, NJ: Pearson.

Miller, R., & Groher, M. (1990). *Medical speech pathology.* Gaithersburg, MD: Aspen.

Montgomery, J. (1992). Implementing collaborative consultation: Perspectives from the field. *Language, Speech, and Hearing Services in Schools, 23,* 363–364.

Moon-Meyer, S. (2004). *Survival guide for the beginning speech-language clinician.* Austin, TX: Pro-Ed.

Moore, M. (1969). Pathological writing. *ASHA, 11,* 535–538.

Moore-Brown, B. (1991). Moving in the direction of change: Thoughts for administrators and speech-language pathologists. *Language, Speech, and Hearing Services in Schools, 22,* 148–149.

National Dissemination Center for Children and Youth with Disabilities. (2008). Retrieved June 10, 2012, from http://www.nichcy.org

National Institute on Deafness and Communication Disorders, 2009.

Nebraska Department of Education. (n.d.). *Measurable annual goals, benchmarks and short-term objectives: What are they?* Retrieved May 16, 2012, from http://www.nde.state.ne.us/SPED/iepproj/develop/mea.html

Nelson, K. (1973). Structure and strategy in learning to talk. *Monographs of the Society for Research in Child Development, 38,* 11–56.

Nelson, K. E., Camarata, S. M., Welsh, J. Butkovsky, L., & Camarata, M. (1996). Effects of imitative and conversational recasting treatment on the acquisition of grammar in children with specific language impairment and younger language-normal children. *Journal of Speech and Hearing Research, 39,* 850–859.

Olswang, L. B., & Bain, B. (1994, September). Data collection: Monitoring children's treatment progress. *American Journal of Speech-Language Pathology,* 55–65.

Owens, R., Metz, D., & Farinella, K., (2011). *Introduction to communication disorders: A life span perspective.* Boston, MA: Allyn & Bacon.

Packer, B. (1995). *Improving writing skills in SLP graduate students through a clinical writing course.* Davie, FL: Nova University ERIC.

Paul, D. (1994). *Clinical record keeping in speech-language pathology for health care and third-party payers.* Updated by Hasselkus, A. (2004). Retrieved June 15, 2012, from http://www.dhs.state.mn.us/main/groups/manuals/documents/pub/dhs16_158228.pdf

Paul, R. (2006). *Language disorders from infancy through adolescence* (3rd ed.). St. Louis, MO: Mosby.

Phillips, D. T., & Mendel, L. L. (2008). Counseling training in communication disorders: A survey of clinical fellows. *Contemporary Issues in Communication Sciences and Disorders, 35,* 44–53.

Ramkissoon, I., & Khan, F. (2003, February 18). Serving multilingual clients with hearing loss: How linguistic diversity affects audiologic management. *ASHA Leader.*

Randolph, D. (2003). Evaluating the professional behaviors of entry-level occupational therapy students. *Journal of Allied Health, 32,* 116–121.

Roseberry-McKibbin, C. (1997). Working with linguistically and culturally diverse clients. In K. Shipley (Ed.), *Interviewing and counseling in communicative disorders: Principles and procedures* (pp. 151–172). Boston, MA: Allyn & Bacon.

Shipley, K. (1997). *Interviewing and counseling in communicative disorders: Principles and procedures.* Boston, MA: Allyn & Bacon.

Shipley, K., & McAfee, J. (2008). *Assessment in speech-language pathology: A resource manual* (4th ed.). Clifton Park, NY: Delmar Learning.

Smit, A. B., Hand, L., Freilinger, J., Bernthal, J., & Bird, A. (1990). The Iowa articulation norms project and its Nebraska reduplication. *Journal of Speech and Hearing Disorders, 55,* 779–798.

Stewart, C., & Cash, W. (2010). *Interviewing: Principles and practices* (13th ed.). Columbus, OH: McGraw-Hill.

Stewart, S., & Gonzalez, L. (2002). Serving a diverse population: The role of speech-language pathology professional preparation programs. *Journal of Allied Health, 31,* 204–213.

Stockman, I. J., Boult, J., & Robinson, G. *Multicultural issues in academic and clinical education.* Retrieved May 15, 2012, from www.asha.org/publications/leader/2004/040720/f040720b.htm

Strunk, W., & White, E. B. (2000). *The elements of style* (4th ed.). Needham Heights, MA: Allyn & Bacon.

Sutherland-Cornett, B. (2006, September 5). Clinical documentation in speech-language pathology: Essential information for successful practice. *ASHA Leader.*

United States Census Bureau. 2011. *Population estimates.* Retrieved April 17, 2012, from http://www.census.gov/popest/data/national/totals/2011/index.html

United States Department of Education. (2005). *A guide to the Individualized Education Program.* Retrieved May 31, 2012, from http://www.ed.gov/parents/needs/speced/iepguide/index.html

Van Riper, C., & Emerick, L. (1989). *Speech correction: An introduction to speech pathology and audiology.* Englewood Cliffs, NJ: Prentice-Hall.

Yarrus, S. (2007, November). *Practical treatment strategies for preschool and school-age children who stutter.* Paper presented at the convention of the American Speech-Language-Hearing Association, Boston, MA.

Zinsser, W. K. (2006). *On writing well.* New York, NY: Harper Collins.

Index